The
Sportsmedicine
Book

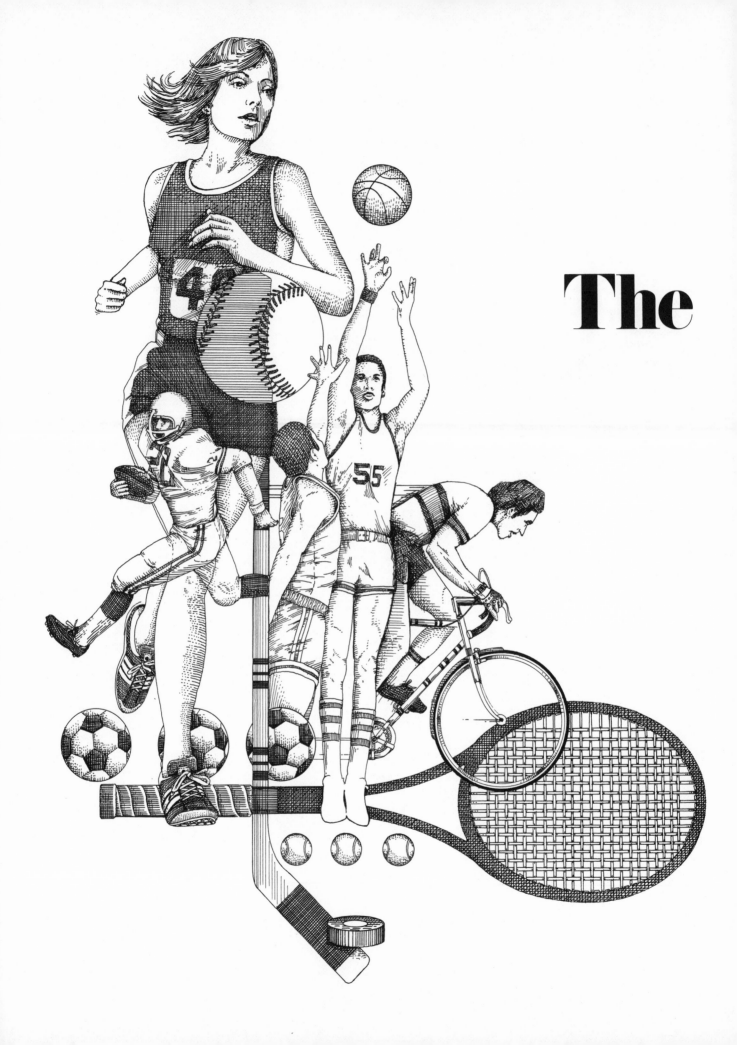

The

Sportsmedicine Book

GABE MIRKIN, M.D.
MARSHALL HOFFMAN

Little, Brown and Company   Boston | Toronto

FIRST EDITION
T11/78

Illustrations by Jeremy Elkin

LIBRARY OF CONGRESS CATALOGING IN PUBLICATION DATA
Mirkin, Gabe.
   The sportsmedicine book.

   Includes index.
   1. Sports medicine.   2. Sports—Physiological
aspects. I. Hoffman, Marshall, joint author.
II. Title. [DNLM: 1. Sport medicine—Popular
works. QT620 M675s]
RC1210.M52   617'.1027   78-14908
   ISBN 0-316-57434-1
   ISBN 0-316-54736-8 pbk.

Designed by Susan Windheim

Published simultaneously in Canada
by Little, Brown & Company (Canada) Limited

PRINTED IN THE UNITED STATES OF AMERICA

To all athletes and fitness enthusiasts.

To Genevieve Young, of Little, Brown and Company, whose knowledge and guidance were major factors in the production of this book.

To our wives, Brigitta U. Hoffman and Irene M. Mirkin.

Acknowledgments

We are indebted to Dr. Ronald Shore, Gabe Mirkin's associate, an editor of the *International Journal of Dermatology* and a former assistant professor at Hahnemann Medical School. He not only saw many of Gabe's patients during the day, but spent hundreds of hours editing the manuscript at night. He also researched and wrote the section on common skin problems of athletes in Chapter 10.

We are indebted to Don H. O'Donoghue, M.D., professor and chairman of the Department of Surgery at the University of Oklahoma Medical School; James A. Nicholas, M.D., director of Orthopaedic Surgery at the Lenox Hill Institute of Sports Medicine and Athletic Training; George Sheehan, M.D., the author of *Running and Being*; and Wayne Leadbetter, M.D., a sportsmedicine physician in Washington, D.C., who took time from their busy schedules to read the manuscript and offer their comments. We are also grateful to the following physicians and scientists for their advice and help with various parts of this book: Robert S. Brown, M.D., Ph.D., University of Virginia; David H. Clarke, Ph.D., exercise physiologist, University of Maryland; C. Carson Conrad, executive director, President's Council on Physical Fitness; David L. Costill, Ph.D., director, Human Performance Laboratory, Ball State University; Fred Goodwin, M.D., National Institute of Mental Health; Gary Gordon, D.P.M., podiatrist, Philadelphia 76ers; David L. Kelley, Ph.D., kinesiologist, University of Maryland; Jack Mahurin, Ph.D., exercise physiologist, Springfield College; William H. Masters, M.D., Washington University in St. Louis; Allan J. Ryan, M.D., the editor of *The Physician and Sportsmedicine*; Ray A. Seelig, editor, "Nutrition Notes"; Roy J. Shephard, M.D., Ph.D., University of Toronto School of Medicine; and Joan Ullyot, M.D., the author of *Women's Running*.

Leading sports figures were generous with their time. We particularly want to thank the following athletes for giving us interviews: Muhammad Ali, Buddy Baker, Larry Brown, Butch Buchholz, Tim Caldwell, Mark Cameron, Robin Campbell, Angel Cordero, Jr., Dan Gable, Roy Hatch, Ron LeFlore, Bobby Moffat, Ken Moore, Al Mottola, Calvin Murphy, Pete Patterson, Kyle Rote, Jr.,

Carmen Salvino, Derek Sanderson, Frank Shorter, Jack Simes, Lee Trevino, and Stephanie Willim.

The following coaches and trainers were extremely helpful with advice, observations, and stories from their own experience: Bob Bauman, trainer, St. Louis Cardinals; Al Cantello, cross country coach, United States Naval Academy; Frank Challant, trainer, Boston Celtics; Gil Clancy, boxing trainer; James R. Counsilman, Ph.D., swimming coach, Indiana University; Tim Davey, trainer, New York Jets; Angelo Dundee, boxing manager and trainer of Muhammad Ali; Brooks Johnson, 1976 Olympic track and field coach; John Lally, trainer, Washington Bullets; Oliver Martin, Olympic cycling coach; Ray Melchiorre, trainer, Buffalo Braves; Gene Monahan, trainer, New York Yankees; Harold Nichols, coach, Iowa State University Wrestling Team; Ed Solotar, swimming coach; Skip Thayer, trainer, Chicago Black Hawks; Greg and Marg Weiss, coaches of gymnastics; Tommy Woodcock, trainer, St. Louis Blues and Superstars.

We are grateful to the athletes, coaches, and trainers of the following teams for interviews: Baltimore Orioles, Boston Celtics, Buffalo Braves, Chicago Black Hawks, Dallas Tornado, Philadelphia Flyers, Philadelphia Phillies, New York Jets, New York Yankees, St. Louis Blues, St. Louis Cardinals, Washington Bullets.

We also want to thank the following runners for their advice and help with this book: Ed Ayres, editor of *Running Times*; Jeff Darman, president of the Road Runners Club of America; David G. Gottlieb, president of the D.C. Road Runners Club; Bob Scharf, former member of the U.S. International Cross Country Team; and Ellen Wessel, president of Moving Comfort, a manufacturer of women's athletic clothing.

Milt Magruder edited our original manuscript and Benjamin Bartolome did our initial artwork.

We would like to give special thanks to Herta Berman, who typed our manuscript over and over again on days, nights, weekends, and holidays.

GABE MIRKIN, M.D., and MARSHALL HOFFMAN
Silver Spring, Maryland

Contents

The
Sportsmedicine
Book

1.

What Is Sportsmedicine?

The Sports Boom

Americans by the millions have been caught up in a new zeal to become fit. A 1977 Gallup poll reveals that almost 50 percent of the adult population, or 55 million Americans, exercise daily. That is almost twice the percentage recorded in 1961.

According to the 1978 Perrier Study on Fitness in America, exercise activities — tennis, football, archery, jogging, swimming, bowling, and others — draw almost 300 million devotees in America. Since there are only 150 million adult Americans, it is obvious that a lot of them take part in more than one sport. And it's a boom that shows no signs of slackening.

Jogging and running have become national pastimes, with 16.5 million people taking to the streets and the parks.

Thirteen and a half million people crowd tennis courts, an increase of 45 percent over a three-year period.

At least three hundred corporate giants provide in-house fitness programs. Overall, according to the National Industrial Recreation Association, company spending on recreation and exercise facilities jumped from two billion dollars in 1975 to three and one-half billion dollars in 1976. The new status symbol in corporate circles is bringing a gym bag or a tennis racket to the office.

More than three hundred marathons — 26.2-mile runs (40 kilometers) — were held in the United States in 1978. Over 4,000 runners officially started the Boston Marathon, the premier long-distance run in the country. Seven thousand men, women, and children entered the Bloomingdale's–Perrier ten-kilometer run around New York City's Central Park, and 5,912 finished.

There are 19.5 million cyclists in the United States. Cycling has become so popular, in fact, that pedal pushers are beginning to get their due: Washington, California, Illinois, and Florida reserve part of their state gasoline taxes to finance bike paths and trails.

No age group is exempt. In one New York gym, four hundred children, some only three months old, are regularly guided through their gymnastic paces. Recently, a seventy-eight-year-old runner finished a twenty-six-mile marathon in San Francisco.

Interest in competitive sports is also at an all-time high. Television has made many athletes as well known as the President of the United States, and in many cases, far better paid.

Muhammad Ali, the former world heavyweight boxing champion, is reportedly the highest-paid American — earning over fifty million dollars in his career to date. For the 6,000 professional athletes in the United States, training and fitness have led to the pot of gold at the end of the rainbow.

Karate	1,500,000
Mountain climbing	1,500,000
Soccer	1,500,000
Squash	1,500,000
Track and field	1,500,000
Wrestling	1,500,000
Judo*	1,500,000
TOTAL:	292,500,000

* Indicates less than a 1% response

BASKETBALL'S TOP EARNERS

David Thompson, Denver Nuggets —	$800,000
Julius ("Dr. J") Erving, Philadelphia 76ers —	$700,000
Pete Maravich, New Orleans Jazz —	$650,000
Kareem Abdul-Jabbar, Los Angeles Lakers —	$600,000
Bill Walton, Portland Trail Blazers —	$550,000

NOTE: All figures are based on published reports. Official figures are not made public.

FOOTBALL'S BIG-MONEY MEN

At least four football players get a quarter of a million dollars or more a year. From published reports, they are:

O. J. Simpson, San Francisco 49ers —	$733,000
Fran Tarkenton, Minnesota Vikings —	$310,000
Larry Csonka, New York Giants —	$300,000
Bob Griese, Miami Dolphins —	$260,000

LEADERS IN BASEBALL'S MONEY GAME

At least eight baseball players are paid a quarter of a million dollars a year or more, according to a press reports.

Vida Blue, San Francisco Giants —	$616,000

Salaries of Professional Athletes

	AVERAGE
Basketball	$125,000
Hockey	$ 95,000
Baseball	$ 73,349
Football	$ 50,000

Reggie Jackson, New York Yankees —	$600,000
Catfish Hunter, New York Yankees —	$560,000
Larry Hisle, Milwaukee Brewers —	$530,000
Oscar Gamble, San Diego Padres —	$475,000
Rich Gossage, New York Yankees —	$460,000
Lyman Bostock, California Angels —	$450,000
Mike Schmidt, Philadelphia Phillies —	$400,000

TOP NATIONAL HOCKEY LEAGUE SALARIES

Ander Hedburg, New York Rangers —	$675,000
Ulf Nilsson, New York Rangers —	$675,000
Gil Perreault, Buffalo Sabres —	$350,000
Brad Park, Boston Bruins —	$265,000
Dennis Potvin, New York Islanders —	$250,000
Marcel Dionne, Los Angeles Kings —	$240,000
Walter Tkaczuk, New York Rangers —	$225,000
Phil Esposito, New York Rangers —	$215,000

OTHER HIGHLY PAID ATHLETES

Muhammad Ali, boxing —	$15,000,000
Jimmy Connors, tennis —	$823,000
Steve Cauthen, horse racing —	$600,000
Chris Evert, tennis —	$503,000
Tom Watson, golf —	$311,000
Jack Nicklaus, golf —	$285,000
Judy Rankin, golf —	$122,000

SOURCE: "Salaries of Professional Athletes" and "Other Highly Paid Athletes" copyright © 1978 Newsday, Inc. All other material courtesy of *The Gazette, The Sporting News*, United Press International, and Rodney Friedman.

Sportsmedicine: An Emerging Science

With increasing participation in both fitness activities and competitive athletics, Americans are eager to learn how their bodies work during exercise and competition. Because I am a physician and a former competitive athlete, and teach a course in sportsmedicine at the University of Maryland, I am often asked questions such as these:

How much exercise do I need?

What is the best exercise for fitness?

Will orthotics relieve my knee pain?

How does carbohydrate packing increase my endurance?

What are the chances of suffering a heart attack during exercise?

How do I prepare myself for an important game?

This book answers these questions and hundreds more. It is a "how-to" book on sportsmedicine, an emerging science that explains how the human body works during physical activity.

Sportsmedicine deals with the physiological, anatomical, psychological, and biochemical effects of exercise, and includes such diverse concerns as training methods, the prevention and treatment of injuries, nutrition, and the effect of weather on the athlete.

It is practiced in part by physiologists, kinesiologists, nurses, podiatrists, physical therapists, trainers, physical educators, chemists, nutritionists, coaches, and athletes, as well as physicians.

Sportsmedicine represents a giant step beyond the time when physicians were concerned only with treating injuries. We are now able to prevent them. I often surprise people who attend my sportsmedicine clinics by picking out those who are most likely to develop pain in their knees, lower back, heels, or soles during exercise. I then teach them how such injuries can be prevented.

I don't mean to imply that sportsmedicine has all the answers. A lot of basic research remains to be done. Solid information backed up by controlled scientific studies just doesn't exist in some areas. For example, I tried to find out how sexual relations affect athletic performance. A computer search of the medical literature failed to reveal a single controlled study.

However, a substantial body of information does exist, and the purpose of this book is to pass it on in practical form to those who need it.

The information in this book comes from years of digesting scientific and medical literature and attending symposia on various aspects of medicine as it relates to physical activity. This research is augmented by interviews with hundreds of athletes, coaches, trainers, scientists, and physicians, and by experiments and observations on my own body during a thirty-year running career.

I have tried to make the information in this book simple and practical, and to concentrate on material that the reader can apply to his or her own activities. As I've said earlier, this is a "how-to" book.

It is a "how-to" book with a message, and the message is one that became obvious to Marshall Hoffman and me after we interviewed hundreds of amateur and professional athletes. The following principles are the theme of the book:

1. *The practices that best prepare the body for fitness and competition are the same ones that lead to health, happiness, and longevity.*

2. *The rules for training, diet, sex, health, and injury prevention apply equally to the weekend exerciser and the professional athlete.* Furthermore, they apply equally to all sports.

The truth of these principles will become obvious to you, too, after you read this book.

Spreading the Word

Nowhere is sportsmedicine practiced more seriously than in East Germany, a tiny country of only 17 million people with a well-established national athletic program. In the 1976 Olympic games, the East Germans won ninety medals. They won forty gold medals, more than were won by American athletes and only a few less than were won by the Russians. One of the main reasons for East Germany's success is the way sportsmedicine information is disseminated to athletes and coaches. All coaches are required to take sportsmedicine courses and to be certified by examination.

According to the President's Commission on Olympic Sports, we know as much about sportsmedicine as any other country is the world. Our problem is that we do not have an adequate system for communicating this information.

I hope that *The Sportsmedicine Book* will be the first step in conveying sportsmedicine information that is now largely unfamiliar to the general public and even, in some cases, to professional athletes. I also want to correct some of the misinformation, misconceptions, and myths frequently believed. That is the purpose of the chapter that follows.

2.

Fifteen Sportsmedicine Myths

Despite the fact that I am a practicing physician and have read everything I could lay my hands on about sports and training, I made some horrible mistakes during my early running career. I used many unscientific training techniques, was a food faddist, and even submitted to unnecessary surgery and cortisone injections. In one race I ran myself into unconsciousness and almost died of a heatstroke.

For years I firmly believed that the athlete who did the most work would be the best. I tried to run a hundred miles a week when my body couldn't take it. I became so weak that I had difficulty getting out of bed. My lymph nodes swelled up all over my body. I thought I had leukemia. It took a major medical checkup, including a lymph node biopsy, to prove me wrong.

At one period, I took such massive doses of vitamin C that my body became dependent on it. I couldn't run as many miles when I stopped taking it.

Three times I broke bones in my feet just from running. I didn't know then that I should have stopped when localized pain increased.

During my running career, I have pulled almost every muscle in my legs. I now know that these injuries could have been prevented.

Now you know how I learned so much about training! Beginners are not the only ones who make mistakes. Some of the greatest athletes in this country are training improperly.

A former coach of the Washington Redskins wouldn't let

his players drink liquids during a pre-season hot-weather scrimmage. Five players, including the starting quarterback, ended up in the hospital with heat exhaustion.

The Chicago Black Hawks trained hard almost every day of the 1976–77 season. Overexertion might explain their poor finish that year.

Greg Luzinski, the Philadelpia Phillies power hitter, was disabled by a pulled hamstring muscle during a recent season. He didn't stretch his muscles daily — the best preventive for muscle pulls.

Million-dollar athletes are advised by the best consultants money can buy. If they fall victim to such mistakes, what are the chances that the 55 million Americans who participate in sports for fun every year won't do the same?

If you understand the science of sports and fitness and are willing to put it to work, you can get the most out of your body and your favorite sport. But first let's clear away some of the mythology and superstition that has grown up around the subject. I have given medical treatment to hundreds of amateur and professional athletes and have talked to hundreds more. During such conversations I have encountered numerous widely held misconceptions. Many of these myths are believed even by top athletes and coaches. Here are some that I run into over and over again.

Myth 1. Athletes Are Born, Not Made

This is just not true. Athletic excellence requires dedication and hard work.

The greatest athletes are those who work hardest without overtraining. Angelo Dundee, who has seen them all, says Muhammad Ali is the hardest-working fighter he has ever seen. Dick Motta, coach of the world champion Washington Bullets basketball team, has to throw his players out of the gym because they practice too much.

Myth 2. You Can Become Fit by Exercising a Few Minutes a Week

A basic element of fitness is the capacity of the heart to do work. This is called cardiovascular fitness.

To achieve cardiovascular fitness, you must push your heartbeat to more than 60 percent of its maximum for at least thirty minutes three times a week. Your maximum is the fastest your heart can beat and still pump blood to your

Dan Gable, the 1972 Olympic gold medalist in wrestling and the most dominant wrestler of all time, forged his determination early. "When I graduated from high school," he says, "I made up my mind to train every day until it was time to retire from competition. From that point, to the Olympics six years later, I gradually increased my workouts to where I was putting in seven hours a day just before the games."

Gable was so conscientious that sometimes he would wake up in the middle of the night to exercise and make up for a missed workout.

body. If you're between the ages of twenty and forty, that level is about 200 beats per minute. That means that you must raise your pulse rate to 120.

If you are a trained athlete and want to maintain a high level of fitness, you must raise your pulse to at least 80 percent of its maximum, or 160 beats per minute, for an extended period.

Since bowling and golf do not raise your heartbeat to these levels, they do not give you cardiovascular fitness.

Myth 3. The More You Train, the More Fit You Become

You can make a mistake by training too hard or by training too much.

The more intensely you train, the less training you can do. Beginners often exercise so vigorously that they become breathless and must cut their workouts short. As a result, they don't get enough exercise to achieve fitness. A good rule of thumb for a beginner: never exercise so hard that you are gasping for air. As your level of fitness improves, you will be able to exercise more vigorously.

When you do too much training, your body breaks down. You become more susceptible to injury and infections. You lose interest in training and are unable to compete at your best.

Amateurs are not the only ones who make this mistake. Mark Cameron, premier weight lifter in America, and Tim Caldwell, a top cross-country skier, both admit that they lost their chances for Olympic medals in 1976 because they overtrained. Now that they've cut their workloads they are performing better than they did during the Olympics.

Myth 4. The Best Way to Improve Your Fitness or Athletic Performance Is to Train Hard Every Day

Every time you exercise vigorously, muscle fibers are slightly damaged and your muscles burn up their fuel and become depleted. You must allow time for your muscles to recover. If you don't, you will be more susceptible to injury.

No great athlete trains as hard as he can every day. You shouldn't either. When preparing for a game, professional football players practice hard only one day a week. Frank Shorter, the former Olympic marathon champion, has days when he runs slower than some high school runners. When playing three times a week, the Philadelphia Flyers, one of

In 1971, Jeff Darman set himself a goal to run a marathon in three hours. "At the time," he says, "I was an unathletic, obese smoker who became short of breath from walking up a flight of stairs." Three years later and fifty pounds lighter, he ran the Boston Marathon in three hours. "Although my time was bettered by seventeen hundred other marathon runners in the United States in that year, it was an achievement for me," says Darman.

Today Jeff is president of the 35,000-member Road Runners Club of America, the premier running organization in the country.

Small But Big

Nate "Tiny" Archibald, past National Basketball Association scoring leader; Gary Player, 1978 winner of three consecutive Professional Golfers Association tournaments including the Masters; and Franklin Jacobs, the 5'8" high-jumper who recently broke the world record when he jumped almost two feet more than his own height, are just three examples of "small" men who have made it "big" in sports. Each of these outstanding athletes has made up with hard work what he lacked in size.

Although the Boston Celtics practice every day they are not playing or flying, hard scrimmages of 45 minutes or more are rare. On game days, the players relax and keep off their feet.

the top teams in professional hockey, often take easy days between games.

Myth 5. If You Attain a High Degree of Fitness, You Will Remain Fit Even with a Layoff

Ridiculous!

Whether you're a runner who can run ten miles with ease or a tennis player who can play three hard sets, you will not be able to handle the same workload after a layoff of even a few weeks.

This is called reversibility, and describes the fact that your muscles — including your heart muscle — quickly lose their ability to utilize oxygen efficiently if they are not stressed constantly. As a result they do not have the same capacity for work after a layoff. In a recent Superstars competition, O. J. Simpson, who normally has amazing stamina, couldn't finish a half-mile run because he was on the banquet circuit and hadn't kept up his training.

Myth 6. You Don't Have to Do Stretching Exercises If You're Fit

Hard exercise shortens muscles and makes them more susceptible to pulls and strains. Therefore, the more physically active you are, the more you need to stretch.

Muhammad Ali stretches for forty-five minutes before each workout. Members of the Buffalo Braves basketball team started stretching five years ago and they haven't experienced any major muscle pulls since.

Myth 7. Exercise Can Harm You Because It Enlarges the Heart

Dr. Paul Dudley White, the eminent Boston heart specialist, said: "Exercise can't hurt a healthy heart."

Exercise puts a moderate stress on your heart, which causes it to become stronger, larger, and more muscular. Heart muscle will *not* turn into fat even if that person stops exercising.

Heart attacks are caused by a failure in the supply of blood to the heart. In an extremely well conditioned person, the arteries supplying the heart with blood are enlarged, and are therefore much less susceptible to clogging or stoppage. This almost guarantees that individual immunity from heart attack.

Clarence DeMar, the great marathon runner who won

When there's no snow on the ground, Tim Caldwell, the outstanding cross-country ski champion, works out 20 hours a week to keep his conditioning. He will cycle 300 miles, jog 15, and roller-ski 50 to 70 miles a week. On off days, he will work out with weights for 45 minutes a day.

Comparative Heart Size in Eleven Types of Athletes

(Based on Herxheimer fractions converted into index numbers)

Tour de France cyclists	24.8
Marathon runners	21.5
Long-distance runners	20.5
Oarsmen	19.3
Boxers	18.9
Short-distance cylists	18.1
Middle-distance runners	18.1
Weight lifters	17.6
Long-distance swimmers	16.4
Sprinters	16.0
Decathlon	15.7

SOURCE: *Towards an Understanding of Health and Physical Education* by Arthur H. Steinhaus, 1963, William C. Brown, Co. Reprinted by permission of Robert A. Steinhaus.

the Boston Marathon seven times, ran almost one hundred miles per week for more than fifty years. If too much exercise could harm a heart, it should have harmed DeMar's. But his heart at seventy was better than that of most thirty-year-olds. The pipes feeding it were three times larger than normal. It would have been almost impossible for DeMar to have had a heart attack.

Myth 8. A Normal Electrocardiogram Means Your Heart Is Healthy and You Can Safely Perform Vigorous Exercise

Not so. A normal resting electrocardiogram means very little. There are reports in the medical literature of people dying of a heart attack immediately after taking a normal electrocardiogram.

A stress electrocardiogram, taken while you are exercising, is another story. If your stress electrocardiogram is normal, you are extremely unlikely to have a conventional heart attack when you exercise.

Myth 9. Vitamin Supplements Improve Fitness and Performance

There is no scientific evidence to support this belief. The average American eats so well that his diet provides all the vitamins he could possibly need.

I took massive doses of vitamins and at one time was convinced I could not perform without them. I finally realized that taking excessive doses of vitamins is unnecessary, and can make you physically and psychologically addicted to them.

Almost every professional team offers vitamin supplements to its players. Why? Don Seeger, the Philadelphia Phillies trainer, explains: "I know that they don't help, but when a hundred-thousand-dollar-a-year athlete asks for a vitamin pill, you don't argue."

Frank Shorter, the former Olympic marathon champion, provides further insight. "I know that vitamins don't work. But after running a hundred and forty miles a week, I would hate to think another athlete might have an advantage over me just because I wasn't taking vitamins."

It is unfortunate that so many athletes waste their money on extra vitamins. Not only are they usually unnecessary, in overdoses they can be harmful.

Athletes Have Bizarre Electrocardiograms

At the 1960 Olympics in Rome, physicians found that more than half of the marathon runners had what they interpreted to be abnormal electrocardiograms.

Dr. George Sheehan once showed a group of heart specialists a series of electrocardiograms without telling them the subjects played football for the New York Giants. The specialists decided that more than 10 percent of the cardiograms were abnormal. But they reversed themselves after Dr. Sheehan disclosed that the tests had been performed on professional athletes.

Wilt Chamberlain, at the peak of his career in the National Basketball Association, once developed such severe abdominal pains that he had to be hospitalized. His electrocardiogram was so abnormal that one doctor mistakenly believed that he had suffered a heart attack. Fortunately, the team physician recognized that Wilt had pancreatitis, an inflammation of the pancreas. Within a short time Wilt was back on the basketball court.

I don't drink or smoke, but I do eat junk food in restaurants. I don't know if I'm getting a balanced diet when I'm traveling. Vitamins are my insurance policy. If I miss something, they give me a second chance. It doesn't matter if I have a urine rich in vitamins.
— CARMEN SALVINO, *a professional bowler for 27 years*

Myth 10. Vitamin B₁₂ Injections Cure Chronic Fatigue

Actually B_{12} injections can only perk up pure vegetarians who have abstained from eating animal products for at least ten years, or persons with pernicious anemia — a rare disease in which this vitamin is not absorbed from food.

Some National Hockey League teams offer their players B_{12} injections after each game, and Muhammad Ali gets a vitamin B_{12} shot two days before a big fight. Such injections have no medical value. Their only benefit is psychological.

A more common cause of chronic fatigue in athletes is potassium deficiency. The treatment: eat large quantities of fruits and vegetables.

Myth 11. Athletes Require More Protein in Their Diet

Muscles are composed of protein, but scientific studies clearly show that protein requirements do not rise significantly with exercise. Hard exercise depletes muscles of muscle sugar (glycogen), not protein.

Greg Weiss, a former Olympic gymnast, believes a high-protein diet helps repair damaged tissue after a hard workout. "I used to make a thick drink out of the protein from powdered milk," he says. "It would shorten my recovery time by a day."

What actually happened? Weiss benefited from the minerals in the drink. The extra protein ended up in his urine.

Myth 12. Steak and Potatoes Are the Best Pre-game or Pre-exercise Meal

Steak ranks as a poor source of immediate energy. Furthermore, the fat in the steak is relatively slow to digest and, if eaten too soon before a game, can actually impair performance.

The best athletic fuel is carbohydrates — found in potatoes, crackers, and bread. Yet almost all of the football and hockey players we interviewed say they are served steak before their games.

I'm a steak-and-potato man.
— DEREK SANDERSON,
Hockey star

Myth 13. You Should Take Salt Tablets to Replace Salt Lost in Sweat

Never take salt tablets! Let your taste buds tell you when to salt your food. If you are low on salt, you will crave salt. Salt tablets bypass your taste buds, which are nature's protection against eating too much salt.

If you get too much salt in your system, you may develop high blood pressure, clots in your bloodstream, or heat exhaustion. Several football players have died in the heat after taking salt tablets. In spite of this, the Boston Celtics, one of the best teams in pro basketball over the years, give out six thousand salt tablets per season. And the Philadelphia Flyers, one of the best teams in hockey, also use salt tablets.

Myth 14. Exercise Should Be Avoided in Cold Weather Because Cold Air Can Freeze Your Lungs

Frozen lung has never been reported in an athlete.

Roy Hatch, one of the top parachutists in the United States, has jumped from a plane at a temperature of 32° F. Falling at 120 to 180 miles per hour, Roy was exposing his body to a temperature of minus 40° F., considering the wind chill factor.

"The only thing that bothers me is my hands," he says.

Myth 15. Amphetamines Improve Athletic Performance

If anything, they hinder it. Amphetamines only make you think you are doing better than you actually are.

In the 1968 Olympics, Japanese weight lifters were widely rumored to have used drugs to overcome their fear of lifting very heavy weights. True, they weren't afraid of the bars, but they couldn't lift them either.

In 1953, forty-one-year-old Gustave Brickner, "the Human Polar Bear," went for a dip in the Monongahela River when the water temperature was 32° F., the air temperature was −18° F., and the wind speed 40 mph. He exposed his body to an equivalent temperature of −85° F., which stands as a record for ice swimming.

3.

The Rewards of Exercise

Why are Americans now turning to exercise in droves?

One reason is that the news is out: Fitness is the new fountain of youth. It is a way to redeem yourself from a life of fast food, beer, and indolence, and it makes you look and feel good.

Research shows that vigorous exercise helps prevent heart attacks, aids weight control, instills a feeling of well-being, and enhances creativity.

Medically, it has been found to help patients with diabetes, ulcers, nervous tension, high blood pressure, back pain, heart disease, depression, varicose veins, recurrent headaches, and menstrual cramps. It cures hangovers, jet lag, constipation, and insomnia.

In diabetes, for example, the reduction of body fat by exercising improves the body's ability to handle sugar.

How Exercise Improves Your Mood

A friend of mine who is a physiologist wanted to write his Ph.D. thesis on what happens when a person stops exercising. He looked for thirty long-term exercisers who would agree to stop exercising for eight weeks. He couldn't find anyone who would volunteer to do so, and had to abandon the study.

People who exercise regularly become physically and

emotionally addicted to exercise. This is called a "positive addiction" because its results are beneficial. Such people are on a natural "high" — are more tranquil, suffer less from tension and anxiety, and are less vulnerable to the stress and irritation of daily life. They are able to concentrate harder, perform better at work or school, and sleep more deeply at night.

My own experience is typical. After seeing myriad patients, I'm beat by 5:00 P.M. My nerves are ajangle. So the first thing I do when I get home is to run.

For the first twenty minutes, I ask myself, "What am I doing out here killing myself?" After thirty minutes, I start to feel euphoric, and my anxieties, tensions, and fears disappear. At forty minutes, ideas flash from the edge of my consciousness. After an hour of continuous motion, colors blend together. Some call it a transcendental peak.

After the run, I'm a new man — no fatigue, no worries — in an exhilarated state that lasts from six to twenty-four hours. Cyclists, wrestlers, swimmers, tennis and basketball players also experience this "high" from exercise.

Numerous clinical studies show that exercise improves mood and imparts a sense of well-being. Herbert de Vries, a professor of physical education at the University of Southern California, tested muscle tension in a group of subjects after half had exercised and half had been given tranquilizers. He found that as little exercise as a fifteen-minute walk is more relaxing than a tranquilizer. Dr. William P. Morgan, a psychologist at the University of Arizona Medical School, finds that exercise leads to decreased anxiety. Tom Cureton, a professor of physical education at the University of Illinois, sent questionnaires to 2,500 regular exercisers, who reported that they have more energy and less tension since they started exercising.

Scientists are unable to explain exactly why or how exercise does this. Some researchers feel that it could be due to increased levels of norepinephrine in the brain. Norepinephrine is a hormone that is necessary for the transmission of brain messages along certain nerves in the body. People who are happy have high levels of norepinephrine in the bloodstream, while those who are depressed have low levels.

Nowhere is this difference more clearly demonstrated than in a psychiatric disorder called manic depressive psychosis, where a patient's mood swings between happiness and depression. During the manic or "high" phase, the patient's level of norepinephrine rises, and during the

It has been said that a five-mile walk will do more good to an unhappy, but otherwise healthy, adult man than all the medicine and psychology in the world. Certainly it is true that, in my own case, nervous stress and strain can be counteracted and even prevented by regular vigorous exercise. It is the best antidote that I know. It is my strong belief that all healthy persons, male and female, should exercise regularly no matter what their ages.

— DR. PAUL DUDLEY WHITE, *heart specialist*

depressive phase, the level of norepinephrine drops sharply.

Scientists don't understand whether norepinephrine is the cause or the result of mood change. Dr. Robert S. Brown of the University of Virginia at Charlottesville and Dr. Fred Goodwin of the National Institute of Mental Health in Bethesda, Maryland, are trying to find out if norepinephrine levels rise with exercise. If the levels do rise, the norepinephrine theory may explain why you feel so good after exercise.

Other theories on how exercise improves your mood:

It increases the blood supply to the brain

With more blood, your brain receives more oxygen. Senile people who are given oxygen often think more clearly and their mood improves. Although there is no hard medical data, exercise may improve mood in a similar fashion.

It decreases the salt level in the brain

Lowering the levels of salt in the brain may improve mood. Dr. Robert Brown has successfully used exercise and diuretics to treat women who become depressed just before their menstrual period. Premenstrual tension and depression can be caused by salt retention due to high hormone levels.

Exercise, by increasing sweat production, and diuretics, by increasing urine production, lower the amount of salt in the body.

Lithium, a new drug used to treat mental disorders, is thought to work in a similar way by driving salt out of the brain cells.

It increases deep sleep

In 1966 Dr. Fred Baekland of the State University of New York was the first to demonstrate scientifically that hard physical exercise promotes deep sleep.

Drs. Colin Shapiro of Johannesburg, South Africa, and R. B. Zloty of the University of Manitoba in Canada, in independent studies, demonstrated that the amount of deep sleep you get is proportional to the daytime energy expenditure. The more you exercise, the deeper you sleep.

People who are free of depression and emotional problems sleep deeply. On the other hand, 85 percent of people who have psychological disturbances have chronic insomnia, according to a study by Dr. Anthony Kales, a professor of psychiatry at Pennsylvania State University. The cause-effect relationship between deep sleep and psychological problems is not clear. However, sleep therapy has been used in European clinics to relieve mental problems. And I have observed that if a depressed person is kept up all night so that he will be exhausted enough to sleep deeply the next day, he wakes up with a markedly improved mood.

It increases your feeling of accomplishment

Dr. Fred Goodwin of the National Institute of Mental Health feels that participation in a regular exercise program gives many people a feeling of accomplishment from successfully completing a difficult task. "Any good feeling about yourself improves your mood," notes Dr. Goodwin.

Dr. Glen Schwarcz, a marathon runner who is head of the running therapy group at St. Elizabeth Hospital in Washington, D.C., says that running helps the therapist as well as the patient. "It is difficult to feel at ease in a closed room with a very sick patient who makes faces and is very angry with you. When you jog, you don't have to look at the patient and you tend to relax. That makes you a more effective therapist. Running also gives the therapist and the patient a camaraderie which couldn't have been achieved any other way. You are doing something together."

Exercise and Mental Disorders

Not only do healthy people benefit from a regular exercise program, but psychiatrists have found that exercise is useful in treating people with varying degrees of mental illness.

Dr. Thaddeus Kostrubala, a San Diego, California, psychiatrist, has treated emotional disorders successfully with jogging. He reports, "I've never experienced this kind of success with psychotherapy. One patient kicked the heroin habit and another, once a paranoid schizophrenic, returned to school and maintained a B average."

In the first controlled study of jogging as a treatment for patients with clinical depression, Dr. John H. Greist, a psychiatrist at the University of Wisconsin, treated them with either running or psychotherapy. Participants completed a widely used symptom checklist that measures degree of depression. After ten weeks, Greist reported that the runners improved greatly while many of the patients on psychotherapy felt no better than before.

Dr. Robert Greenwood of the Menninger Foundation in Topeka, Kansas, offers another explanation. Abnormalities of the mind are often accompanied by abnormalities of muscle function. That's why emotionally disturbed people often make bizarre movements with their bodies. Treatment of mental and physical disorders go hand in hand.

Some form of exercise can aid the neurotic and even the most severe psychotic.

A Love Affair with the Heart

I've always believed that exercise strengthens the heart and helps prevent heart attacks, and this belief is supported by numerous scientific studies and surveys. Because of my conviction, I started the Run For Your Life program in 1963 in Baltimore, Maryland. It is now a national program where people of all ages and abilities run for fun and fitness. Awards are given for participation, not excellence. The program is sponsored by the Road Runners Club of America.

To attract runners, I offered a trophy to everyone who completed the two-mile course in twenty-two minutes.

One participant was Walter Korpman, a forty-year-old, six-foot-two, 180 pounder who formerly had been a heavy smoker. With a burst of speed, Korpman finished two seconds under the twenty-two-minute time limit. A half hour after the run, I found Walter lying on the ground, still gasping for air. Terrified, I envisioned a newspaper headline: "Man Dies in Run For Your Life Program."

Korpman admitted that he had trained for only two weeks before the race. Months later I found out that he had previously had a heart attack. Physicians at the time were advising patients who had a history of heart attack to avoid strenuous exercise.

Walter eventually developed into one of the country's best master runners (over forty years of age). He could run a mile in 4:55 and two miles in 10:30.

Walter did not become one of the 700,000 Americans killed each year by heart attacks, the greatest killer in America today.

Drs. Ralph Paffenbarger of the Stanford Medical School and Jere Morris of the London School of Hygiene and Tropical Medicine demonstrated that exercise is associated with a lower incidence of heart attacks.

What is a heart attack?

The heart is nourished by coronary arteries on its outer surface. When fat is deposited on the inner surfaces of these arteries, a plaque forms, which may obstruct the flow of blood. If the plaque builds up on an artery to the point

Your Heart

The heart, which is about the size of a man's fist, is the finest pump known to humankind. In the average adult, it beats 40 million times a year, and more than 2.8 billion times in a lifetime. In a person of average size, it pumps 4,300 gallons of blood daily through 60,000 miles of blood vessels.

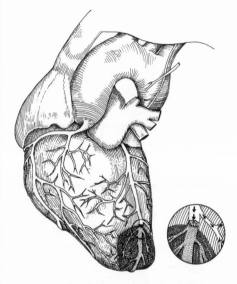

A conventional heart attack: A fat plaque obstructs the blood supply and the part of the heart muscle supplied by that artery dies.

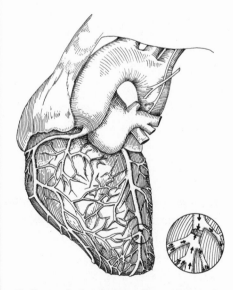

Collateral circulation: Several arteries supply blood to the same area.

where the blood supply is cut off, the part of the heart muscle fed by that artery dies. If a large part of the heart muscle dies, the heart can no longer pump blood through the body, so the body dies.

Heart-attack pain ranges from a dull pressure to a sharp, cutting sensation that is like being stuck with a knife. It can occur either at rest or with exertion. It usually arises in the left side of the chest, but can occur anywhere in the chest or upper abdomen. Classically, the pain begins in the left side of the chest and radiates down the left arm, and is brought on by exertion. However, most chest pains people experience are caused by muscle spasms or gas in the intestinal tract and are not associated with the heart.

How does exercise help?

It enlarges all the coronary arteries which feed the heart.

It increases collateral (auxiliary) circulation so that more than one blood vessel will supply a given area of the heart. If the blood supply becomes blocked in one artery, blood from another will nourish the area and prevent a heart attack.

It lowers the concentration of fat in the blood. Fatty plaques obstruct the coronary arteries, causing heart attacks. More than ten years ago, John Holloszy, a medical researcher in St. Louis, demonstrated that blood levels of fats, called triglycerides, can be lowered by vigorous activity. Lowering blood fat levels decreases the tendency to form fat plaques that clog the blood vessels.

It teaches the heart to extract oxygen from the blood more efficiently.

It lowers blood pressure.

Will exercise bring on a heart attack?

According to Dr. Roy J. Shephard, a professor of preventive medicine at the University of Toronto, the chance that a heart attack will occur in a normal man during one-half hour of heavy exercise is one in 5 million. In a normal woman, the chance is one in 17 million.

Dr. Kenneth Cooper, author of *Aerobics,* reports seeing only two heart complications in the last six years among 2,276 exercisers who, in total, walked or ran three-quarters of a million miles at his Institute of Aerobics Research. That works out to only one complication for every 93,409 hours of participation, or 391,097 miles covered. The two who experienced heart problems recovered fully and are still running today.

Exercise and heart disease

Years ago many physicians mistakenly equated the athlete's heart to that of a person with congestive heart failure. Both hearts are large, but for different reasons. The congestive heart appears large because the muscle is stretched with fluid. The athlete's heart is large because it is muscular. Paavo Nurmi, who won nine gold medals for Finland in long-distance running, had a muscular heart three times normal size.

Whenever a middle-aged person calls me about starting an exercise program, I'm always careful to ask about any history of chest pain. Many times such individuals tell me that they have had chest pains, but their physicians performed a resting electrocardiogram and reassured them that their hearts were normal. Resting electrocardiograms often fail to detect blocked coronary arteries.

The most reliable test to predict susceptibility to heart attacks is the stress electrocardiogram, taken while a person exercises. A stress electrocardiogram can be obtained from physicians in private practice or from any large medical center or medical school. Dr. Myrvin Ellestad of Long Beach, California, found that 40 percent of his patients who showed abnormalities in a stress electrocardiogram had a heart attack within five years. However, other studies indicate that a poor result on a stress electrocardiogram can be improved after the patient undergoes a medically supervised exercise program.

Not only is exercise recommended to prevent heart attacks, it is also used by some doctors to treat victims of heart attacks.

Dr. Terrence Cavanaugh of Toronto, Canada, brought eight post-heart-attack victims to compete in the Boston Marathon. Seven of them finished and none suffered adverse effects. Dr. Jack Scaff, a Hawaii-based cardiologist, encourages his heart patients to run in the Honolulu Marathon. Drs. Noel Nequin of Chicago, Illinois, Joe

	ATHLETIC HEART 50 BEATS PER MINUTE	AVERAGE HEART 75 BEATS PER MINUTE	DIFFERENCE
1 minute	50	75	25
1 hour	3,000	4,500	1,500
1 day	72,000	108,000	36,000
1 month	2,160,000	3,240,000	1,080,000
1 year	25,920,000	38,880,000	12,960,000
Lifetime (72 years)	1,866,240,000	2,799,360,000	933,120,000

The Athletic Heart Beats Better

Because the athlete's heart is so muscular, it can pump the same amount of blood with 50 beats per minute that the average heart pumps with 75 beats per minute. Thus, the athlete's heart will beat 13 million fewer times per year. It works less, rests more, and consequently takes a much longer time to wear out.

Rogers of Trenton, Michigan, Pat Gorman of Washington, D.C., and Herman Hellerstein of Cleveland, Ohio, are among many cardiologists who treat heart-attack victims with jogging. All of these doctors' patients are under strict medical supervision. If you have a history of chest pain or heart disease, a doctor's guidance is mandatory for any exercise program you may undertake.

Why don't all medical authorities agree that exercise helps to prevent heart attacks?

It is almost impossible to design a study that controls all the associated factors — high blood pressure, excess weight, smoking, etc. However, Dr. Tom Bassler, a physician and a marathoner, has been unable to document a single case of heart attack caused by fatty plaques in a marathoner. Does this mean that running marathons gives absolute immunity from heart attacks? Not necessarily, but the incidence of heart attacks in such individuals must be extremely low.

Marathoners do avoid other risks associated with coronary disease. They usually don't smoke. They aren't overweight, and they have lower blood pressures and blood fat levels. They usually keep regular hours and tend to be relaxed and free from tension, probably due to their running.

Indeed, Dr. Arthur Mollen, a physician and runner, couldn't find a single coronary risk factor in a study of marathoners.

Dr. Cooper found that the more fit an athlete is, the less likely he is to have any of the coronary risk factors.

When a person starts exercising, he usually changes his life-style. It creates a sort of chicken-or-the-egg controversy: Is it the exercise or the change of life-style that helps prevent heart attacks? Perhaps it is both.

Exercise Takes Off Pounds

Are you losing the battle against creeping obesity? Exercising for as little as thirty minutes a day will help you shed unwanted fat.

In my own case, I lost forty pounds in the first six months of my running program. I didn't reduce my food intake — if anything, I ate more.

Dr. Kenneth Cooper tells about a patient who had angina, a heart pain brought on by even slight exercise. Angina is caused by a partial blockage of one or more of the blood vessels supplying the heart. Because his angina was so severe, the patient became depressed and decided to commit suicide by running himself to death. He felt his insurance company would not interpret a running accident as a suicide. So he ran as far as he could until he collapsed of exhaustion. To his amazement, he survived. The next night he ran again and covered a greater distance before he collapsed. Night after night he ran, until he could run two miles without stopping. At this point, his angina disappeared. He became a regular jogger and lost his interest in suicide.

Energy Expenditure by a 150-Pound Person in Various Activities*

ACTIVITY	CALORIES PER HOUR
A. Rest and Light Activity	50–200
Lying down or sleeping	80
Sitting	100
Driving an automobile	120
Standing	140
Domestic work	180
(continued)	

Runner's World magazine surveyed eighty runners — all past forty years of age. All showed weight loss, averaging thirteen pounds, compared to their pre-running days. None had gained weight.

Dr. Michael Pollock of Wake Forest University examined thirty-two men who averaged forty-seven years of age and had been jogging for several years. The tests showed their body fat was 10 to 15 percent below levels found in the overall population of the same age group.

Many people are discouraged from exercising when they find out that in order to lose a single pound they must run 4 hours, ice skate 9 hours, play volleyball 10 hours, or walk 17 hours. But you don't need to do all that exercise at one time. If you spread these hours over a week or two, you will have lost a substantial amount of weight at the end of a year.

To have an effective weight reduction program, you *must* exercise. Dieting without exercise is doomed to failure because:

You will lose muscle as well as fat. In 1915, Dr. F. G. Benedict of the Massachusetts General Hospital demonstrated that 25 percent of weight reduction through dietary restriction is due to loss of muscle tissue. Thus, after you lose weight, you will have less muscle. If and when you start to take in more calories than you burn, your weight gain will be entirely fat. The result: You will have more fat on your body than you had originally, and you will have proportionately more fat and less muscle in your body. With less muscle to carry your added weight, you will become even more inactive and gain even more weight.

You are not likely to keep the weight off. Becoming and remaining thin requires great dedication. People who are not willing to exercise are not making a full commitment and usually are not willing to change their life-style. As a result, they are more likely to go back to their old eating habits.

You're not as hungry

You become hungry when your blood sugar level drops precipitously. When you exercise regularly, your blood sugar level doesn't fluctuate much. Here's the reason: During exercise, your body mobilizes fat into the bloodstream. Your muscles use proportionately more fat and don't take as much sugar out of the bloodstream.

B. Moderate Activity	200–350
Bicycling (5½ mph)	210
Walking (2½ mph)	210
Gardening	220
Canoeing (2½ mph)	230
Golf	250
Lawn mowing (power mower)	250
Bowling	270
Lawn mowing (hand mower)	270
Fencing	300
Rowboating (2½ mph)	300
Swiming (¼ mph)	300
Walking (3¾ mph)	300
Badminton	350
Horseback riding (trotting)	350
Square dancing	350
Volleyball	350
Roller skating	350

C. Vigorous Activity	over 350
Table tennis	360
Ditch digging (hand shovel)	400
Ice skating (10 mph)	400
Wood chopping or sawing	400
Tennis	420
Water skiing	480
Hill climbing (100 ft. per hr.)	490
Skiing (10 mph)	600
Squash and handball	600
Bicycling (13 mph)	660
Scull rowing (race)	840
Running (10 mph)	900

*The standards represent a compromise between those proposed by the British Medical Association (1950), Christensen (1953), and Wells, Balke, and Van Fossan (1956). Where available, actual measured values have been used; for other values a "best guess" was made.

SOURCE: Robert E. Johnson, M.D., Ph.D., Professor of Biology, Knox College, Coordinator, Knox Rush Medical Program, Scientific Consultant, Department of Medicine, Presbyterian St. Lukes Hospital, Chicago.

Your body absorbs fewer calories

When you exercise, food passes through your intestinal tract quickly. In medical terms, peristalsis increases. Marathon runners find that a meal can pass through their systems in as little as four to six hours. The transit time for most people is usually twelve to twenty-four hours.

Scientists are unable to explain increased motility in the intestinal tract. But it happens. That's why athletes have massive and frequent bowel movements. One theory is that exercise causes the body to release increased amounts of magnesium into the intestinal tract. Magnesium is commonly known as the cathartic Epsom salts.

For several hours after you stop exercising, your body continues to burn calories

Dr. Herbert de Vries has shown that the increased metabolic rate that occurs *after exercise* in an average exerciser can result in a five-pound weight loss in one year.

Exercise may promote weight loss in obese people by another mechanism. Captain Robert Simon of the United States Air Force reports in the *Journal of the American Medical Association* that many obese people eat to ward off depression. Because exercise improves mood, it can be used as an effective therapy to treat both the cause — depression — and the result — obesity.

For the first three weeks or more of an exercise program you may not lose a single pound. Don't become discouraged. Several studies have shown that when you start to break down fat, you retain water. However, after a few weeks, you'll urinate out the extra fluid and lose weight quickly, sometimes as much as three to five pounds in a day.

How quickly you lose weight depends on the difference between the amount of food your body absorbs and the amount you burn. To lose one pound of fat, you must have a negative caloric balance of 3,500 calories.

If you are an average male, you take in 3,000 calories per day. If you run thirty minutes a day, you will burn 450 calories; if you don't increase your food intake, you will lose a pound of fat in about a week.

The most effective exercises are those that are vigorous and sustained. That's why running, cycling, swimming, and aerobic dancing are best. Bowling, golf, and walking, on the other hand, are less effective.

Oliver Martin, the 1976 United States Olympic bicycling coach, told us that champion bicycle racers have frequent bowel movements. "They eat so much that when they are not on their bikes, they are on the toilet."

A Testimonial

Six years ago, I brought my son to Dr. Mirkin to be checked for asthma. I knew that Dr. Mirkin was a runner and I casually remarked that I was a runner too. Dr. Mirkin looked me up and down. "You can't be a runner because you're too fat," he said without scorn.

It was true that I was heavy — 240 pounds on my 6'2" frame — but I was running five miles a week.

I left his office with a cured son and a sick ego.

During the next six months, I increased my mileage from five to a hundred miles a week. My weight dropped from 240 to 170 pounds and my waist size decreased from 44 to 32 inches. I thought of myself as an efficient running machine.

Expecting his hearty congratulations, I went back to Dr. Mirkin. "You are still seven pounds overweight," he remarked.

I was so shocked that I went to the University of Maryland for body fat tests. Dr. Mirkin was right. The tests showed that I had 6½ pounds of extra body weight.

While running, I was attacked and severely beaten in February 1977. For six months I couldn't run. Even though I wasn't eating any more, my weight jumped up to 200 pounds. Now that I'm running again — from eight to twelve miles a day — my weight has decreased to 180 pounds.
— DAVID G. GOTTLIEB
   President, D.C. Road Runners Club

General Well-Being

Seven medical experts were asked by the President's Council on Physical Fitness and Sports to rate fourteen sports and exercises on a scale of 0 to 3, indicating their effectiveness in promoting general well-being. Thus, a rating of 21 for an exercise means it was viewed as most beneficial, since each of the experts gave it a score of 3.

	WEIGHT CONTROL	MUSCLE DEFINITION	DIGESTION	SLEEP	TOTAL
Jogging	21	14	13	16	64
Bicycling	20	15	12	15	62
Swimming	15	14	13	16	58
Skating (ice or roller)	17	14	11	15	57
Skiing — Cross Country	17	12	12	15	56
Handball/Squash	19	11	13	12	55
Basketball	19	13	10	12	54
Calisthenics	12	18	11	12	53
Tennis	16	13	12	11	52
Skiing — Downhill	15	14	9	12	50
Walking	13	11	11	14	49
Softball	7	5	8	7	27
Golf	6	6	7	6	25
Bowling	5	5	7	6	23

SOURCE: The President's Council on Physical Fitness and Sports.

Losing Inches

When you exercise, you turn fat into energy and build muscle. Muscle is much heavier than fat. That's why you will lose inches long before you lose pounds. You will be delighted to learn that the areas you will reduce are the areas in which you store fat: the abdomen, thighs, buttocks, and hips.

The loss of body fat should interest women especially, because 25 percent of the average woman's weight is fat, compared to 15 percent for the average man. As a woman ages, the percentage of her body fat increases. By exercising she will become more compact and attractive and lose those unsightly bulges.

Have you seen a vibrating machine that has a belt that is

Joan Ullyot, M.D., who became an international marathon runner at thirty-three, says: "In my five years of running even though I haven't lost any weight, my pants size has gone from 14 to 10."

placed around your buttocks? It's supposed to reduce your hips by shaking them and is based on an erroneous principle called spot reduction. All it does is shake up your bladder and give you a headache. It doesn't make any difference what part of your body you exercise. The only way to rid yourself of fat is to burn more calories than you take in. Then your fat will disappear from the places it is stored.

Big, Ugly Muscles Don't Happen

It amazes me that so many women are worried that exercise will build large, ugly muscles. It doesn't happen. Ice skater Dorothy Hamill and gymnast Olga Korbut have sleek, well-formed muscles. To develop large, bulky muscles, you have to do resistance exercises such as weight lifting. Rhythmic exercises such as aerobic dancing, running, swimming, and bicycling form long muscles and a firm, attractive figure.

4.

The Universal Rules of Training

Dr. A. Rogozkin, the physician for the Russian 1976 Olympic teams, predicted that "in the next Olympic games those countries with the best science behind their athletes will be the big winners."

Training today is so scientific that an athlete, trainer, or coach who ignores or fails to understand certain immutable rules may be throwing away an Olympic gold medal, a Super Bowl, a Stanley Cup, or a World Series pennant.

In interviewing hundreds of professional and amateur athletes, coaches, and trainers, we've discovered that even some of the best athletes don't fully understand all of the basic principles of training.

Many professional athletes, even though they may be earning more than $100,000 a year, do not observe the rules and thus are not getting the maximum performance out of their bodies.

Here are the five Universal Rules of Training:

Specificity: Your training must be specific. To perfect a sport skill, you must practice that skill, using your muscles in the same manner you would when you compete.

Hard and Easy Days: You must schedule hard days for intensive workouts and easy days for recovery.

Training and Overtaining: To improve maximally, you must increase your body's capacity by increasing its workload, but not beyond its limits.

Background and Peaking: Your training should begin with a background period in which you progressively increase your workload. Shortly before the time when you want to be at your best, you should begin a peaking period in which you decrease the amount of your workload and increase its intensity.

Reversibility: Even if you have worked for a lifetime staying in top physical shape, you cannot take off more than a few weeks before you lose your conditioning.

Specificity

People often ask me if participating in different sports will improve their performance in their own sport. The answer is "no." The best training for a sport is to practice that sport.

Training for any sport requires work on a combination of the following factors:

Coordination: Use your muscles *in the same manner* you will use them in competition.

Speed: Use your muscles *at the same speed* or faster than you will use them in competition.

Strength: Use your muscles *against resistance* in the same manner you will use them in competition.

Coordination

Coordination is a complex process. The eyes are the first link in the system: they send the images you see along a pathway of nerves to your brain. The brain interprets the signal, decides which muscles should contract and how hard and fast the contractions should be, and sends out messages along another network of nerves. For every muscle that contracts, there is an opposing muscle that relaxes, and the brain coordinates the movements of every muscle in the body simultaneously. The entire process takes a fraction of a second.

When you dive into a pool or hit a tennis ball with your racket, every one of your five hundred muscles receives instructions from the brain. That's why you can spend a lifetime improving coordination.

Practice improves coordination in two ways. First, your brain interprets messages faster. Second, the brain sends more specific directions to the muscle, so that the motion is more precise and efficient.

How Athletes Develop and Maintain Coordination

After twenty-seven years as a professional bowler, Carmen Salvino is still one of the best. He bowls 100 to 150 games a week.

"Mentally, I bowl 365 days a year," Salvino says. "Physically, I miss only 50 days a year.

"Eight months ago I broke a toe. My doctor ordered me to rest, but I knew that if I did, I would lose some of my coordination. Because my foot hurt too much to bowl, I would walk up to the line and swing my arm as if I had a ball in my hand."

Ron LeFlore, all-star outfielder for the Detroit Tigers, keeps a bat at home to swing 50 to 100 times a day in off-season. "This helps to keep my hands and arms in coordination with my eyes," says LeFlore. "I always want to keep that sense of rhythm."

Kyle Rote, Jr., All-Star soccer player and a three-time winner of the Superstar competition, says: "I set challenging goals for myself in every workout. For example, I won't leave a workout until I can kick the soccer ball perfectly into the air 50 straight times."

Speed

To be fast in competition, you must train fast in practice.

Here's the reason:

Your muscles are composed of at least two different types of fibers — slow twitch fibers and fast twitch fibers. The slow twitch fibers are for endurance. Because of their rich blood supply, they appear red under a microscope. The fast twitch fibers are for speed and strength. Because they have a limited blood supply, they appear white under the microscope.

The ratio of fast twitch to slow twitch fibers in a muscle is determined before birth. There is nothing an athlete can do to change this ratio. Good athletes in endurance sports tend to be endowed with a greater percentage of slow twitch fibers, while great sprinters tend to be endowed with a greater percentage of fast twitch fibers.

However, you can maximize the performance of the fibers you have through training. For example, slow running develops slow twitch fibers, just as fast running develops fast twitch fibers.

Doc Counsilman, our country's greatest swimming coach, says: "You have to swim fast in training to swim fast in races. We did muscle biopsy studies and found that the fast twitch fibers that make you swim fast are developed by speed swimming. That's why my swimmers swim fast almost every day."

Years ago marathon runners trained only by running long distances. Now they know that to race at a fast pace, they must train at a fast pace. Frank Shorter runs at a five-minute-mile pace in marathon races, but he can't possibly run twenty-six miles that fast every day when he is training. Therefore, he uses the interval technique. Three times a week he runs short distances at a very fast pace — close to four minutes per mile.

Weight lifters also need to develop speed. How fast they start the bar moving determines how much they can lift. That's why champion weight lifters perform sets of ten repeats moving the bar as fast as they can.

Training is so specific that a person may be able to train his arms to move very fast and still not be able to move his legs very fast. For example, a pitcher may be able to throw a ball at speeds greater than ninety miles per hour and still be the slowest runner on the team.

While Johnny Bench has enough arm speed to hit home runs in the Superstars competition, his swimming speed was so slow that he barely made it across the pool.

Strength

You develop strong muscles by making them lift heavy weights, but a traditional weight-lifting program is not always the answer. You must also use your muscles in the same manner that you will use them when you compete. Therefore, the best way to become strong for a sport is to perform that sport against resistance. "Against resistance" means using heavier equipment to do the same thing you will do in competition.

For a baseball player, it's swinging a weighted bat; for a golfer, it's swinging a weighted club. (However, heavier bats and clubs also slow down your swing. To guard against this, baseball players and golfers should also swing light bats and clubs very fast to maintain their speed.)

O. J. Simpson and many other running backs lift leg weights to develop strength in their legs and lower bodies because this gives them power to break tackles.

A runner needs strong arms since a runner's arms help him run. But runners don't need to press heavy weights above their heads. It won't help them because they don't run with their hands over their heads. If they want strong arms, they should use pulleys arranged so that they pull heavy weights with the same motion they use when they run.

Hard and Easy Days

Top athletes don't perform the same workout each day. You shouldn't either. You should vary your workouts and follow the hard–easy principle.

Hard days

Hard days are those days when you put a nearly all-out effort into your workout. Improvement comes from these hard days, when the body is stressed. Stress refers to the intensity an athlete puts into his workout, not the amount of time spent working out. However, the body must be stressed for a minimum amount of time in order for the improvement to take place. This time will vary with the sport and your condition, but the intensity of the exercise usually must be enough to make you pant and sweat, and increase your heart rate. In medical terms, a beginner

When Weight Lifting Doesn't Work

"Muhammad Ali got strong from hitting heavy bags and sparring with big guys, not heavy weight lifting," says Angelo Dundee, his manager. "Hitting a heavy bag developed the same muscles he uses to fight. Lifting heavy weights could never be that specific."

Butch Buchholz, the commissioner of World Team Tennis, tried weight lifting when he was a top tennis player, but gave it up. His reason: "It didn't make me as strong as playing tennis several hours a day. I found that hitting the ball hard made me stronger for tennis."

How Top Athletes Vary Their Workouts

Ken Moore, twice an Olympic marathoner, runs hard only three days a week. On the other four days, he runs easily.

Mark Cameron, America's top weight lifter, lifts heavy weights two or three times a week, but never on consecutive days. On the other days, he stretches and lifts lighter weights.

stresses himself when his pulse goes over 60 percent of its maximum rate for several minutes. That's about 120 beats per minute for the average man or woman. A trained athlete in top condition may have a hard day when his pulse goes over 80 percent of its maximum rate for an extended period of time.

Easy days

Stressing the body has a price — minor injuries to muscles that require time to heal. That's why you must work easy days into your training program.

You will benefit from a heavy workout only if you allow your muscles time to recover. If your muscles are stressed before they recover, they deteriorate.

Why do your muscles need to recover from a heavy workout?

Medical scientists give three reasons:

Muscle fiber is damaged by hard exercise and, like any other tissue in the body, requires healing time proportionate to the amount of injury.

Muscle fuel, called glycogen, is used up. It takes the body ten hours to ten days to replenish it.

Potassium, a mineral released from the muscle cell to control heat, is also depleted. It takes up to forty-eight hours to restore the supply.

By measuring the level of certain enzymes in the bloodstream, scientists can now measure the degree of muscle damage from exercise. These chemicals usually are found in the muscles but are released into the bloodstream during a heavy workout.

Recovery time

A recovery period or an easy day does not mean an athlete does nothing. He must still work out, but at a lower level of intensity. Performing at a relaxed pace hastens recovery.

Coaches and athletes have argued for years about an optimum recovery period. Even now coaches can't agree on the proper length of time between hard workouts. Most athletes we interviewed allow a forty-eight-hour recovery period from hard workouts or games.

Doc Counsilman prefers a twenty-four-hour recovery period. His swimmers work out twice every day — once hard, the other easy. His reasoning: "The swimmer's body

A Hard Day

	HEART RATE FOR A HARD DAY	MAXIMUM HEART RATE
Beginner between the ages of 20 and 40	120	200
Person over 60	96	160
A fit person	135	200
Athlete	at least 160	200

What Top Athletes Do on Their Easy Days

"On my easy days I run twenty miles at a relaxed pace," says Frank Shorter, a marathoner with two Olympic medals to his credit.

Oliver Martin, the United States Olympic cycling coach, recommends "five to six hours of easy pedaling on recovery days."

Dan Gable, the 1972 gold medalist in wrestling, wrestles continuously for forty minutes on hard days. On easy days, he cuts the mat time to twenty minutes.

The National Basketball Association's Buffalo Braves had a poor season in 1976–77. One possible reason: The team played or practiced for three months before the players were given even one Sunday off.

The Chicago Black Hawks hockey team finished poorly during a recent season. Says a team member: "We did hard workouts every day so we didn't really have any easy days."

Before the 1972 Olympics, Gerry Lindgren, a 10,000-meter runner who had made the 1968 team while still in high school, tried to run 300 miles a week. He never took an easy day and he didn't even make it to the trials. His body couldn't recover from his training schedule and it broke down.

is horizontal in the water — and the heart doesn't pump against gravity. Buoyancy relieves some of the overload on muscles. Thus swimmers can recover faster than runners."

Recovery from competition usually takes even longer than recovery from heavy workouts. Frank Shorter needs two weeks to recover completely from a marathon. Mark Cameron says he requires seven to ten days to overcome fully the effects of a weight-lifting meet.

Professional football teams have also adopted the hard–easy technique. The New York Jets are a good example. Sunday usually is game day — their hard day. On Monday, the players review game films, do stretching exercises and, to work up a sweat, run a light drill. Tuesday is a day off for all players. Wednesday is game-plan day — with the hardest and most physical practice of the week. There's a moderate workout on Thursday; a very easy day Friday. On Saturday, players polish up their game plan and travel if the game is out of town. Sunday is back to all-out football.

Training and Overtraining

Johnny Weissmuller, who later became famous as Tarzan of the movies, won the 1924 Olympic 400-meter freestyle in 5 minutes, 4 seconds. In the same event in 1976, Petra Thumer, an East German schoolgirl, swam almost one minute faster.

Tom Hicks won the 1904 Olympic marathon in 3 hours and 28 minutes. Today, that time wouldn't even qualify him for the Boston Marathon. The present world record for that event is eighty minutes faster.

The fantastic improvement in athletic performance has been brought about by athletes who have literally extended the frontiers of the human body by increasing its workload prodigiously. Athletes are now routinely doing things that were assumed to be beyond human capacity just a few decades ago.

However, there is an upper limit to the amount of work even the most highly conditioned body can perform. There is a fine line between work and overwork. Sports history is full of stories of athletes who overtrained themselves out of great careers.

Derek Clayton, the world record holder in the marathon,

A History of Increasing Workloads

Paavo Nurmi dominated long-distance running in the 1920s because he trained with short, fast bursts of speed interspersed with slow jogs. This enabled Nurmi to run more fast miles than any other competitor in his time. No published records are available, but Nurmi probably ran more than 50 fast miles a week. Prior to Nurmi, distance runners ran time trials three times a week.

After World War II, Emil Zatopek of Czechoslovakia further increased the workload and won all three distance events in the 1956 Olympics. His method was to run 12 to 36 miles in workouts, alternating fast and slow runs, called intervals. In all, he would run more than 70 fast miles a week.

Percy Cerutty of Australia and Arthur Lydiard of New Zealand paved the way to further improvement when they recognized that short fast bursts limit the workload by using up more muscle sugar and oxygen. Their approach was to fun fairly fast over long distances and this boosted the training load to more than 100 miles a week.

and Dave Bedford of England, the former world record holder in the 10,000-meter run, both ran two hundred miles a week in training. Their careers were ended by injuries before either won an Olympic championship, because they didn't recognize the signs of the overwork syndrome.

In 1936, Dr. Hans Selye, a physician at McGill University in Montreal, demonstrated that if rats were stressed and then allowed to recover, they became stronger. Rats that were stressed again before they recovered became weaker. Rats that were not stressed didn't improve.

I had learned about Dr. Selye's work on stress and overwork in medical school. But before I could apply his principles to my training, I suffered the syndrome myself.

The same signs and symptoms that Dr. Selye found in overworked rats appear in overtrained athletes.

If you are always tired and suffer from frequent colds and injuries, you are probably overtraining.

These are the other signs of overwork:

IN THE MUSCLES
Persistent soreness and stiffness in the muscles, joints, and tendons
Heavy-leggedness

EMOTIONAL SYMPTOMS
Loss of interest in training
Nervousness
Depression
"I don't care" attitude
Inability to relax
A drop in academic or work performance

BODY WARNING SIGNS
Headache
Loss of appetite
Unexplained drop in athletic performance
Fatigue and sluggishness
Loss of weight
Swelling of lymph nodes in the neck, groin, and armpit
Constipation or diarrhea
Absence of menstruation

Overtraining is a serious problem among beginners, amateurs, and professional athletes. Beginners usually do too much for their out-of-shape bodies to handle, become injured or fatigued, and quit their program. Seasoned amateur or professional athletes who overwork are frequently injured and always dragging. The result: less than their best performance.

Large Workloads Take Tremendous Dedication

"After my tenth-place finish in the 1962 Olympics, I decided to become an Olympic champion," says Bruce Jenner, the 1976 decathlon champion. "For the next four years, I trained eight hours every day. I took off only one day — Christmas — and I felt guilty."

Angelo Dundee, who has managed many champions, calls Muhammad Ali "the hardest-working fighter I've ever seen. He outworks everybody. He is always jogging, sparring, punching light and heavy bags, watching fight films. He sometimes sneaks out at 3:00 in the morning to run. If you run with him, he will try to run you into the ground. He either trains or sleeps.

"Behind all that talk and poetry is a very hard-working man who likes preparing for a fight."

George Young, four-time Olympic distance runner, never took a day off. "Whenever I looked out the window and saw a driving snowstorm," he explains, "I would tell myself that the Russians are out there running."

Mark Cameron, the best weight lifter this side of the Iron Curtain, describes the sacrifices made by members of the United States weight lifting squad: "Two guys lost their jobs, one guy lost his wife, I lost a year of graduate school, and everyone lost money."

For at least fifty years, athletes and coaches have relied on the resting morning pulse to pick up signs of overtraining. The procedure is simple. When the athlete first opens his eyes, he takes his pulse for sixty seconds. If it is more than seven beats per minute faster than usual, he either takes the day off or cuts back in his workouts.

The East Germans, with the most science-oriented sports program in the world, perform measurements of enzyme levels in the blood. When muscles are damaged, the enzymes are released from the muscle and their concentration rises in the bloodstream. Athletes with higher than normal enzyme counts in the blood are told to decrease their training.

Dr. Lloyd Drake of New Zealand does hemoglobin levels — an indicator of red blood cells — on John Walker, a world record holder in the mile. If his hemoglobin level starts to fall, Walker cuts back on his workouts. Most experts express skepticism about this procedure.

Doc Counsilman doesn't believe in the blood tests, either. "I've performed white blood cell counts as early as two decades ago," he says. "I don't put much faith in them. I feel that their value lies in the fact that you can tell an athlete that his blood is normal and that he or she is okay to swim."

I agree with Counsilman. Good coaches can tell when their athletes are doing too much.

Background and Peaking

Great champions prepare their bodies so they will perform at their very best on the day of an important competition. This is achieved by using a technique called "peaking" — decreasing the volume and increasing the intensity of training as the time of a competition approaches. Peaking is used by runners, rowers, cyclists, swimmers, boxers, and other athletes who compete in sports requiring strength and endurance.

In peaking periods, an athlete performs much less work but at a higher degree of intensity. Training is specific. During peaking, a weight lifter lifts heavier weights with fewer repeats. A swimmer swims thirty miles a week instead of sixty, but swims them faster.

On the other hand, background training is the body-building process — to improve strength, endurance, and

Signs of Overtraining

Swimming coach Ed Solotar can tell when his swimmers overtrain. "When they can't keep up, I send them home."

Jim McKenzie, the trainer for the Philadelphia Flyers, reports that superstar Bobby Clarke runs into an overtraining syndrome from playing 40 to 45 minutes a game. The average playing time for hockey players is 20 to 25 minutes. "When Clarke is tired," McKenzie says, "I can see that he has a slower reaction time and is more susceptible to injury."

Stephanie Willim, formerly one of the top gymnasts in America, starts to cry when she overworks.

Mark Cameron, America's top weight lifter, tells us that when he overtrains, his joints begin to ache.

Cross-country skier Tim Caldwell describes the overwork syndrome this way: "I become tired and heavy-legged. I get colds easily and I don't like to train."

Marathoner Frank Shorter says, "When I overtrain, lymph nodes swell up in my groin."

A study at the Tokyo Olympics showed that the athletes had more infections than their coaches, presumably because they were training hard while their coaches were only advising.

skill over the long term. In the background phase of training, competitive athletes perform large workloads, which thicken their tendons and ligaments, improve heart function and circulation, and teach their muscles to extract oxygen more efficiently from the bloodstream.

One coach that I interviewed compared background training to putting money in the bank. Peaking, he said, was spending the money you saved in the background period.

No matter how great your athletic ability, you can't hold a peak for more than six to eight weeks. The reasons:

> Competition and intense workouts sap the body of its strength. Recovery takes longer. The more intense the competition or workout, the easier it will be to injure yourself.
>
> Because you can't keep up your workloads, your body is deconditioning.

Athletes who compete in strength and endurance events must learn to alternate between background and peaking training. Most of the year must be spent in background training, concentrating on increasing workloads. About a month before competition, the athlete should start decreasing the volume and increasing the intensity.

Peakers

Some athletes peak only for the Olympics — once every four years.

Lasse Viren, a double gold medal winner at 5,000- and 10,000-meter runs in two Olympics, ran forty-eight races in 1971 and lost many of them. "I can only peak for six weeks," he explains. "After that, I have to go back and pile up the miles [background training]." After the 1972 Olympics, he was beaten frequently. By the 1976 Olympics, Viren was again unbeatable.

Al Oerter won four gold medals in the discus over a sixteen-year period. Between Olympics, he often lost.

Sports history is full of peakers and nonpeakers. Ron Clarke, considered by many to be one of the world's greatest distance runners, raced anyone, anywhere, anytime. During his career he seldom went three weeks without a race. Clarke held the world record for almost every distance from two to ten miles. Yet he never won a major race. Because he trained the same all year, less

How to Peak

Weight lifter Mark Cameron says, "I didn't fully understand background and peaking until a few years ago. I lifted heavy almost up to competition. Now I know better."

He takes his last heavy workout three weeks before an important competition. Then, in each succeeding workout he lifts less total weight but attempts to lift to a heavier top weight.

"In the peaking training period, I will lift 90 percent of top weight," Cameron explains. "For example, I will clean and jerk 420 pounds in practice. I feel that the pressure of a competition gets my adrenalin flowing and I can lift at least 10 percent more than in practice."

capable runners who peaked beat him in the Olympics and British Commonwealth games.

Luzins, Von Ruden, and Winzenreid — the three best 800-meter runners in 1972, winning virtually every race at that distance — had raced so much the prior winter that they were "bankrupt" in the Olympic trials and failed to make the U.S. team.

Team sports — soccer, football, baseball, basketball, and hockey — use the training camp for their background period. The teams play so frequently during the season that they can't train as much as in training camp. Thus, the entire season is a modified peaking period.

Billy Martin, manager of the 1977 World Series champion New York Yankees, does not drive his players hard in spring training. Gene Monahan, the Yankee trainer, explains Martin's reasoning this way: "If he worked the players too hard in spring training, how would they get through the next six months of playing almost every day?"

Peaking Too Early

If you are competing in an individual sport and preparing for a specific meet, you must be careful not to reach your peak too early. Because of the high intensity of training in the peak period, you can maintain peak performance for only a limited time. If you try to prolong the peaking period, you will experience the overwork syndrome and your performance will deteriorate.

There are a number of causes for peaking too early, among them:

Starting your peaking period too soon
Entering too many competitions during the peaking period
Performing more intense training than your body can handle
Not cutting back your workload when you increase your intensity

Here is an example of peaking too early.

A high-school miler wants to run a 4:30 mile for the state championship. He runs the following times on successive weeks: 4:48, 4:42, 4:34, and then 4:41. His drop in performance means that he has peaked too early and he must resume slow background training. If he continues to train by running very fast intervals, his racing performance will deteriorate further.

Weight lifters can also peak too early. For instance, a

The Best Peakers

One of the all-time best peakers — both physically and mentally — is Mark Spitz, winner of seven gold medals at the 1972 Olympics.

"He had the best mind for competition of any athlete I've ever known," says Doc Counsilman, who has produced many Olympic champions. "Mark could do anything that he set his mind on. My job was to set his goals high enough and convince him that he could get there."

At the 1972 Olympics, Spitz was exhausted after he won his fifth gold medal. He had finished second to an Australian swimmer in a heat in the 100-meter butterfly. Spitz was discouraged and wanted to drop out of the competition.

"Look at the Australian swimmer," Counsilman recalls telling Spitz. "They had to drag him out of the pool."

Although Spitz's pulse was elevated, Counsilman told Spitz his pulse was OK and "that shows that you are not tired."

"Really, coach?" a wide-eyed Spitz responded. A few minutes later, in reply to a reporter's question, Spitz said, "I feel great."

Because of a psychological peak, Spitz won not only the butterfly but a relay race as well, to earn seven gold medals in one Olympics — a feat never equaled in the history of Olympic competition.

Another great peaker was Peter Snell, a distance runner from New Zealand. In two Olympiads, he never was seriously challenged. In the 1964 Olympics, he decisively won seven middle-distance races in nine days.

Six weeks earlier, he couldn't break four minutes for the mile. His time wouldn't even have qualified him for the Olympics. Arthur Lydiard, Snell's coach who also coached New Zea- *(continued)*

weight lifter wants to clean and jerk 350 pounds. On successive weekends, he cleans and jerks to a top weight of 315, 325, 325, 335, and then 310. At this point he will have to resume lifting to lighter top weights for a week or two. If he insists on training with near top weights, his performance will deteriorate further.

Reversibility

Whether you are a world-class athlete or a housewife swimming for exercise, it takes only three to four weeks for your body to lose its conditioning. It doesn't matter if you have been training all your life. Scientists call it reversibility.

Scientists do not completely understand why reversibility occurs so quickly. John Holloszy of Washington University in St. Louis, Missouri, has shown that muscles, if they are not stressed constantly, rapidly lose some of their ability to use oxygen efficiently. That means reversibility sets in quickly for aerobic endurance sports such as swimming, cycling, long-distance running, and cross-country skiing which require the muscles to use oxygen over an extended period of time.

Reversibility sets in at a slower pace for weight lifters and sprinters. To perform their events, they don't need oxygen. They don't lose strength or speed until their muscles get smaller from lack of use.

Even with reversibility creeping in, sprinters can still run at top speed, but they won't be able to run repeat heats at the same speed. The same applies to weight lifters. They may still be able to lift top weights but cannot do it repeatedly.

Besides a drop in performance, how do you know that you're suffering from reversibility?

> You will be short of breath. After a two-week layoff, you will find yourself gasping for air at the same pace that you were comfortable with before your layoff. This is because your muscles are having problems utilizing oxygen.
> Your muscles will be sore. No one knows why, but the most widely accepted theory is that during reversibility, your muscle fibers become smaller. Smaller fibers are weaker, tear more easily, and take longer to heal. It's the tearing that causes the soreness.

land's Olympic team, planned it that way. He knew that a runner cannot remain in peak form for more than eight weeks and had Snell doing background training at that time. Six weeks later Snell proved to be the best middle-distance runner in the world.

Fighting Reversibility

Most top athletes never get out of shape. Calvin Murphy is one of the smallest players in the National Basketball League at 5'9" and 165 pounds. In off-season, he runs a baton-twirling school — and had 117 students in his 1977 class. "I'm running around more in the off-season than during the basketball season," says Murphy. "I give basketball clinics; I cycle all the time; twirling makes me use the muscles in my chest and arms. And I jump rope to keep my timing. When I report to training camp, I'm about twenty days away from my peak condition."

Doc Counsilman gives his competitive swimmers only two three-week vacations a year.

Lee Trevino, the Canadian Open and Colonial National champion in 1977 and one of the leading money winners in professional golf for the past ten years, plays almost every day in the off-season.

Because of reversibility, it takes far less time and effort to get out of shape than it does to become fit. Larry Brown, when playing with the Washington Redskins, stopped training when the football season ended. He admits that within three or four weeks his fitness disappeared. "That's why I suffered so much in training camp," explains Brown. "I'd kill myself getting back into shape."

5.

How Your Muscles Work

Endurance

Endurance is a basic element in the performance of any sport. In competition such as cross-country skiing, marathons, and long-distance cycling it is the key factor in determining who wins. That is why these sports are called "endurance sports."

Endurance can be increased by training designed to improve:

The capacity of your muscles to store and burn muscle fuel

The ability of your system to deliver oxygen to the muscle—muscles need oxygen to burn fuel efficiently

Muscle Fuel

Food components are divided into three groups:

Protein. Never a source of immediate energy and a poor source of energy during exercise. It is the building block for tissues in the body. The body has no way to store extra protein.

Fat. A secondary source of energy especially during the latter stages of endurance sports. Fat is stored in the muscles, under the skin, and around the inner organs.

Carbohydrates. The primary fuel for exercise. Your body stores carbohydrates in the muscles and in the liver in the form of glycogen.

The Factors That Limit Muscular Endurance

Loss of muscle glycogen — the primary fuel of the muscle

Loss of fat reserves — a secondary fuel for the muscle

Low level of blood sugar, called hypoglycemia (blood sugar is a secondary source of muscle fuel)

Lack of oxygen, called hypoxia

Accumulation of lactic acid, a breakdown product of exercising without oxygen

Heat buildup in the muscles, called hyperthermia

During exercise a muscle cannot take in enough energy-producing food products to replace what is being used up. This means that if you start out in a competition with a greater amount of glycogen stored in your muscles, you will have greater endurance.

"Hitting the Wall"

What happens when a muscle runs out to glycogen? That muscle will become uncoordinated and begin to hurt. It's called "hitting the wall," a very common phenomenon during endurance competitions. "Hitting the wall" is particularly prevalent during marathons that take place during warm weather. Exercise in the heat uses up more glycogen than exercise in mild or cold weather. Most novice marathoners "hit the wall" before twenty miles. That's why the stragglers at the end of a marathon look as if they have been on the Bataan Death March.

Once glycogen is bound in a muscle, it stays in that muscle until it is burned. It cannot migrate from one muscle to another. That is why the muscle that is being exercised the most will run out of glycogen first. For example, a boxer's arms may run out of glycogen before his legs do.

With willpower, you can keep on going after "hitting the wall," and your muscles will burn fat, blood sugar, and finally their own tissue. When this happens, every movement becomes extremely painful.

Depletion

Depletion is a training program used by endurance athletes that is based on the fact that your muscles will learn to store more glycogen if their supply is used up frequently. The more glycogen the muscle can store, the longer it can work.

In 1939 Erik Christenson, a Swedish physiologist, demonstrated that endurance depends on the amount of glycogen bound in the muscle before exercise. Further studies showed that a scientist could predict how long a muscle could exercise by measuring the glycogen inside it. In 1966–67, Jonas Bergstrom, another Swedish physiologist, fed various diets to athletes and measured the amount

In the 1963 Boston Marathon, two Ethiopian runners streaked through the streets of Beantown's suburbs, setting new records at every checkpoint. At the nineteen-mile mark, they were more than three minutes ahead of the field.

Suddenly their legs weakened and then went dead. Their long graceful strides became uncoordinated. Abbebe Bekila and Mamo Wolde, both Olympic champions, stumbled across the finish line, in fifth and thirteenth places. They had "hit the wall."

Duncan MacDonald, a U.S. Olympic distance runner, was asked by a reporter why he dropped back after leading in the 1977 Honolulu Marathon for fifteen miles. MacDonald replied: "I was running along fine until I hit the wall." The reporter asked him if he had hurt himself.

Every time I've run more than twenty-two miles continuously I've hit the wall. It creeps up on me and then suddenly my legs go dead. My legs hurt all over, but the most severe pain is in my thighs. My body tells me to slow down, but by concentrating on each step, I can maintain my pace. My only thought is to reach the finish line. At this point in the race, I've promised myself that I will never run a marathon again.

Immediately after crossing the finish, I start to feel better. The intense pain disappears and even though it hurts to walk, I'm at peace with the world. My mental anguish disappears and I can't remember the misery of hitting the wall. I look forward to my next marathon.

— GABE MIRKIN, M.D.

of glycogen inside the muscles. He demonstrated that if an athlete exercised his muscles to exhaustion to deplete his glycogen and then ate a carbohydrate-rich diet, he could triple the amount of glycogen his muscles could hold and the workload they could do.

The amount of exercise you must perform to deplete your muscles varies widely, and depends on your level of training. The novice jogger may deplete at four miles, while a topnotch marathon runner may not deplete until he has run over twenty miles. The time it takes to deplete your muscles is also extremely variable, so much so that the same person may have different depletion times on different occasions.

You can tell that your muscles are depleting when they start to ache and you have difficulty coordinating them. To deplete fully, you must use them for some time after the discomfort sets in — about five to ten minutes for the average runner.

There is an upper limit to the amount of glycogen any muscle can store, and even athletes in peak condition will undergo the ultimate depletion and "hit the wall" at some point. For a top marathon runner, this point will come at about twenty-two to twenty-five miles; for a cross-country skier, sixty miles, and for a champion cyclist, perhaps at seventy to one hundred miles.

When I start to get back in shape each summer, my muscles ache all the time. But as I get into condition, my muscles stop hurting.
— LARRY BROWN,
former All-Pro back
for the Washington Redskins

When the bell rang for the fifteenth round in the thrilla in Manila against the gorilla, my arms were so tired that I could barely raise them above my trunks.
— MUHAMMAD ALI

Burning Fat

Frequent depletion will also teach your muscles to burn a greater percentage of fat during all stages of exercise, and thereby spare muscle glycogen. Burning fat with muscle glycogen is up to thirteen times more efficient than burning glycogen alone. Scientists call this "burning fat on the flame of glycogen."

It's like a sailboat with two power sources: gas for an outboard motor, and wind for the sail. When the wind blows, gas is saved.

Carbohydrate Packing

For years scientists have known that carbohydrates are the primary fuel for hard exercise. But until recently they were

Ron Hill, one of the top marathon runners in the world, has been running for more than twenty years. During the last eight, he's practiced carbohydrate packing. "Before 1969," he says, "I would tire at eighteen miles. I don't train any differently from the way I trained then, but now I go twenty-four miles before I hit the wall."

unable to use this knowledge to devise a diet that would significantly improve endurance.

The method of carbohydrate packing now used by most endurance athletes was devised in 1967 by Per-Olof Åstrand and Eric Hultman, two Swedish scientists and recognized authorities on sportsmedicine.

Six days prior to an event for which he is training, the athlete exercises to exhaustion the muscles to be used in competition. Then for the three days he limits his carbohydrate intake and eats mostly protein and fat — meats, fish, poultry, eggs, unprocessed cheese, and butter. Fruits contain carbohydrates and should be limited. This keeps the sugar content of the exercised muscles low. This is the depletion phase.

During the next three days, just prior to the event, he eats many small meals that are rich in carbohydrates. This forces the muscles to bind extraordinary amounts of carbohydrates, which are then available as muscle fuel during the stress of the event. This is the loading phase.

The amazing number of new world records in endurance events may in part be due to this practice.

In 1971, Jonas Karlsson and Bengt Saltin found that in a 30-kilometer race (18.6 miles), runners improved their times 7.7 minutes with carbohydrate packing. This figure is remarkably close to Paul Slovic's 1975 report of an 11-minute improvement in marathon runners' times using Åstrand's carbohydrate-packing technique.

Although virtually all marathon runners agree that you should stock up on carbohydrates before a race, they do not all agree that the depletion phase is necessary. Frank Shorter, the former Olympic marathon champion, does not follow the carbohydrate depletion phase because he depletes so frequently in practice. Evidently his body dosen't require it.

Cyclists don't do it either. "Before a race, cyclists have to practice six or seven hours daily," says Olympian Jack Simes. "If they don't have any carbos in their system, they ain't gonna make it."

Dangers

Even for endurance athletes in top physical shape, carbohydrate packing can be fraught with potential problems. *It can possibly cause death.* The severe carbohydrate restriction during the depletion phase of the loading process can cause ketosis. This is an accumulation of toxic substances in the blood, and can lead to kidney damage and

1,530 Carbohydrate Depletion Diet Plan
(For the Three Days Prior to Carbohydrate Loading)

BREAKFAST	*calories*
eggs, 2	150
coffee, 1 cup	10
orange juice, ½ cup (contains carbohydrate)	50

LUNCH	
salmon patty, 4 oz.	200
lettuce and tomato salad (tomato has carbohydrate)	75
tea	10

SNACK	
celery, 3 stalks	50
bacon, 2 strips	100
unprocessed cheese, 1 oz.	100

DINNER	
chicken, 1 leg	200
chicken, 1 breast	210
leafy green salad (contains a small amount of carbohydrate)	75
apple, 1 medium (contains a small amount of carbohydrate)	75

SNACK	
yogurt made from skim milk, 1 cup	120
carrot, 3 sticks	75
cauliflower, 1 cup	30
Total:	1,530

personality changes. This danger can be minimized by drinking a lot of fluid — at least eight glasses a day. Older athletes and people with kidney and liver diseases are particularly susceptible to these side effects and should not attempt the depletion phase.

In 1973, I reported in the *Journal of the American Medical Association* a case of a forty-year-old man who developed chest pain and an abnormal electrocardiogram while undergoing carbohydrate packing. This case may have been due to the ingestion of massive amounts of carbohydrates during the loading process. Another explanation may be that his abnormal electrocardiogram and chest pain resulted from the deposition of a very large amount of glycogen in the heart muscle itself. Gorging can severely raise the fat level in the blood. It is not necessary to gorge.

Prostatitis — a swelling of the prostate gland accompanied by painful urination — is another potential complication and is probably due to inadequate fluid intake during carbohydrate packing. During this process, the athlete should drink far more liquids than usual . . . at least eight glasses a day.

Potassium deficiency can accompany the loading phase. When the muscle is enlarged by increased amounts of glycogen, more potassium is required. Potassium is the primary mineral inside the muscle cell. Varied fruits, which are a rich source of potassium, should be eaten during the packing phase to prevent any deficiency.

Dr. William Banks of the University of Pennsylvania showed that during the loading phase following depletion muscle cells may break down and release myoglobin into the bloodstream. Myoglobin, a large protein, can damage the kidney.

The athlete also should recognize that the extra sugar in his muscles will make his legs feel heavy.

Because all long-term effects of repeated supercompensation are not known, Åstrand's method should not be attempted more than two or three times a year. To understand carbohydrate packing better, a depository for listing side effects has been established and reports can be sent to Dr. Ben Londeree, Director, Exercise Physiology Lab, 36 Rothwell, University of Missouri, Columbia, Missouri 65201.

Even with its side effects and shortcomings, a carefully controlled program of carbohydrate packing can help the performance of endurance athletes such as the long-distance rower, runner, cycler, skier, or channel swimmer.

Carbohydrate Packing Diet
(4,040 Calories)
(For the Three Days before Competition)

BREAKFAST	*calories*
orange juice, 1 glass	100
oatmeal with raisins, 4 bowls	400
toast, 4 pieces	240
butter, 2 tablespoons	100
coffee, 2 cups	20

SNACK	
oranges, 2	140
banana, 1	130

LUNCH	
tomato juice, 1 glass	100
cheese and tomato sandwiches, 2	400

SNACK	
Swiss cheese sandwich	250
apple, 1	75
pear, 1	75

DINNER	
chicken, 1 leg	200
chicken, 1 breast	210
bread, 5 pieces	300
vegetable salad (no dressing)	75
spaghetti, 3 cups	600
tea, 1 cup	10
potatoes, 2	240

SNACK	
peanut butter sandwich	175
orange, 1	70
banana, 1	130
Total:	4,040

Carbohydrates for the nonendurance athlete

What about athletes such as tennis players, football, or basketball players? Carbohydrate packing in nonendurance events — less than thirty minutes of continuous exercise — has minimal effect on an athlete's performance. Athletes in events not requiring prolonged endurance should simply eat a diet rich in carbohydrates the day before the event.

Bonking

Endurance athletes suffer from another type of fuel-loss syndrome called "bonking," which has a different cause from "hitting the wall." In medical terms, the body runs out of liver glycogen. Glycogen is also stored in the liver, where it becomes blood sugar, the primary source of energy for the brain. Within a few minutes of running out of liver glycogen, the blood sugar level drops and the brain cannot function properly. I remember one novice runner who had "bonked" and took a swing at me when I tried to pick him up after he fell at the twenty-first mile of a marathon.

The symptoms of "bonking" are dizziness, shakiness, confusion, lack of coordination, and cold sweat.

If you eat immediately, you can recover from a bonk. But if you can't get food immediately, you won't be able to finish the race.

Taking nourishment during competition prevents bonking. Skier Tim Caldwell eats and drinks every fifteen minutes to forestall it.

There are important physiological differences between "hitting the wall" and "bonking." When a runner, skier, or fighter "hits the wall," he runs our of muscle glycogen and he can't come back. "Bonking" is running out of liver glycogen, which can be replaced immediately by eating.

It's possible to "hit the wall" and "bonk" at the same time. I've done it.

When I was twenty-eight years old I entered a twenty-mile race in Leonardtown, Maryland. I had not run a single practice run of more than six miles. In those days, it wasn't in vogue to load carbohydrates and my precompetition meal was a meager portion of spaghetti.

At fourteen miles, my legs became so heavy I was barely able to shuffle along. I had "hit the wall" — but I kept on moving, slowly. At eighteen miles, I suddenly broke out in a cold sweat; my hands started to shake and I was

Possible Side Effects of Carbohydrate Packing

POSSIBLE SIDE EFFECTS OF THE DEPLETION PHASE

Nausea	Headache
Muscle weakness	Irritability
Tiredness	

POSSIBLE SIDE EFFECTS OF THE PACKING PHASE

Heart pain	Tiredness
Muscle pain	Muscle weakness
Painful urination	Heavy arms
Bloody urine	or legs

During a 160-mile bicycle race, an Australian rider missed his food pickup. He broke out in a cold sweat and started to shake. He then became weak, dizzy, and confused; his eyes began to bulge; he was "bonking." He asked the other riders in the breakaway for some food. They refused. Only when he paid $75 would they give him three cheese sandwiches. After eating them, his strength returned and he won the race and the prize money.

— JACK SIMES,
three-time Olympic cyclist

As long as my riders can get some food into them immediately, they can "bonk" and come back many times in a race. Except when they are approaching a steep climb, I tell them to reach back into their bag and take food every fifteen minutes during the entire race.

— OLIVER MARTIN,
the U.S. Olympic cycling coach

starving — symptoms of low blood sugar. It was a "bonk."

Fortunately, my wife was following in the car. Feebly I motioned her to give me something to eat. All she had was two pounds of cookies, which I quickly devoured. I finished the race by moving each leg with my hands.

Thus, during the race, I recovered from the "bonk," but not from "hitting the wall." My legs were sore for two weeks.

Oxygen

Muscle glycogen and fat are converted into energy in the muscle by burning. To burn these fuels efficiently, oxygen is needed. Oxygen is delivered to the muscles through the bloodstream by the red blood cells.

Roy J. Shephard, a famous physician and researcher at the University of Toronto, has shown that the crucial factors in oxygen utilization are the ability of the heart to push the blood to the muscles and the ability of the muscles to extract the oxygen from the blood.

You can improve your oxygen utilization through exercise. By training you can:

Strengthen your heart muscle so that it can pump a greater volume of blood with each beat

Enlarge your arteries so more blood can flow through them

Increase the number of your red blood cells so your blood's oxygen-carrying capacity is increased

Increase the rate at which enzymes in your muscles pick up oxygen from the blood

The VO_2 max

The maximum ability of your body to deliver oxygen to your muscles is limited by your genetic makeup and varies substantially from individual to individual. The peak rate at which the body can take in and use oxygen is called the VO_2 max (max = maximum, V = volume, O_2 = oxygen).

Don Lash, who held the world record in the mile in the 1930s, and Jim Ryun and Kip Keino, world record holders in the same distance in the 1970s, have the same VO_2 max — 81. Yet both Keino and Ryun could run the mile sixteen seconds faster than Lash.

What is the reason for this? It is because Ryun and

"Bonking" rarely occurs in trained runners, even in 100-mile races. One memorable exception was the case of Ed Winrow, a national champion distance runner. He tells this story about a 1967 marathon.

"I thought I was going well until the twentieth mile. I was running up a hill, and a lady pushing a baby carriage passed me from behind. Some officials tried to pull me out of the race, but I fought them off. Finally they convinced me to quit."

Dave Costill, a Ball State University professor, measured the heart volume of the late Steve Prefontaine. It was 40 percent larger than that of the average American of the same age, height, and weight.

VO_2 Max of Top Distance Runners

RUNNERS	VO_2 MAX AS MEASURED IN CC/KG × MINUTES	HEART RATE MAXIMUM (BEATS PER MINUTE)
Barry Brown	77.9	195
Ted Castenada	76.8	196
Jeff Galloway	73.0	196
Paul Geis	79.9	186
Don Kardong	77.4	198
Mike Manley	76.1	198
Ken Moore	74.2	192
Philip Ndoo	80.8	194
Russ Pate	76.9	204
*Steve Prefontaine	84.4	210
Frank Shorter	71.3	195
Gary Tuttle	82.7	214
Ron Wayne	72.9	192
Untrained males	38.4	191

*Now deceased

SOURCE: Dr. David Costill, Ball State University

Keino can compete closer to their VO_2 max for a longer time. Modern-day athletes have assumed workloads unheard of just a few decades ago, and thereby have increased their endurance.

That is why world records in endurance sports are constantly improving. Take marathoner Ron Daws, whose heart has a maximum rate of 187 beats per minute. No matter what he does, his heart cannot beat faster. He has reached the top of his VO_2 max. But he can maintain his pulse rate at 180 beats per minute, or 95 percent of his maximum, for more than two hours and twenty-five minutes, the time it took him to run an entire marathon.

Dr. Cyril Wyndham of South Africa has shown that world records in endurance events depend on an athlete's ability to use more than 80 percent of his VO_2 max during the entire competition.

Derek Clayton, world record holder in the marathon, can run at 86 percent of the maximum amount of his oxygen capacity (VO_2 max) throughout an entire marathon.

Can the administration of oxygen help an athlete?

Yes, but only during hard competition.

When a football, basketball, or soccer player comes out of a game, it is useless to give him oxygen because at rest and immediately after hard exercise, even when he may be sucking for air, the blood vessels leading away from his lungs are 98 percent saturated with oxygen.

However, during exercise, the amount of oxygen in the lungs diminishes and giving oxygen improves performance. According to Herbert A. de Vries, professor of exercise physiology at the University of Southern California, 66 percent oxygen is the most effective concentration to administer during competition. Breathing 100 percent oxygen can make you dizzy.

Lactic Acid

When glycogen is burned, it is broken down to a chemical called pyruvate. If there is enough oxygen available, pyruvate converts to the end products carbon dioxide and water, which are blown off from the lungs. However, if there's not enough oxygen in the muscles, pyruvate converts to lactic acid, which builds up in the muscle and then overflows into the bloodstream. Lactic acid impedes

Why You Need Oxygen

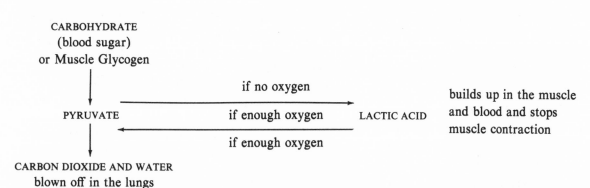

CARBOHYDRATE
(blood sugar)
or Muscle Glycogen

PYRUVATE   if no oxygen   LACTIC ACID   builds up in the muscle
    if enough oxygen   and blood and stops
    if enough oxygen   muscle contraction

CARBON DIOXIDE AND WATER
blown off in the lungs

muscle contractions and makes it increasingly difficult for muscles to move. As a result, you feel fatigue. A high level of lactic acid will eventually stop the muscle from contracting altogether. When this happens, you lose control over the muscle, and it becomes increasingly painful and may cramp.

A shortage of oxygen, called an "oxygen debt," is signaled when you begin to breathe hard and pant during exertion. This is the way your body tries to take in more air. Every athlete incurs an oxygen debt and builds up some amount of lactic acid during competition, when he is working full out. However, trained muscles can continue to contract with a much higher amount of lactic acid.

As soon as oxygen becomes available, lactic acid converts back to pyruvate and then to carbon dioxide and water.

Exercise or competing with enough oxygen to fire muscle fuel is called "exercising aerobically" or "paying as you go." If you are a novice and can run two miles in sixteen minutes without becoming breathless, that is an aerobic pace for you. But if you try to run the distance in fourteen minutes, you begin to pant, build up lactic acid, and become fatigued. This is called exercising anaerobically.

You should understand that if you work so intensely that you run up an oxygen debt and build up lactic acid, you will tire quickly and limit the amount of work you can perform.

Blood Doping

In the early 1970s, Bjorn Ekbloom, a Swedish physiologist, developed a controversial method for improving endurance, called blood doping.

When I started to run a year ago, I would gasp for breath at a twelve-minute-mile pace. Now I don't become breathless until I run at an eight-minute-mile pace.

— MARSHALL HOFFMAN

About a month before competition, Ekbloom withdraws 20 percent of an athlete's blood, then siphons off the fluid and refrigerates the red blood cells. The athlete's body quickly makes new blood and blood levels are back to normal within three weeks.

Seven days before competition, the stored red blood cells are reinfused into the athlete's body, raising the concentration of red blood cells far above normal and increasing the bloodstream's oxygen-carrying capacity.

Ekbloom claims that "blood doping" increases an athlete's performance by 3 to 5 percent.

However, most physiologists do not believe that method improves performance.

"Although there is no doubt that the blood carries more oxygen, it is much thicker," points out Dave Costill, a leading exercise physiologist at Ball State University. "The increased viscosity of the blood makes it more difficult for the heart to pump, especially through the small veins and capillaries. What you gain in increased oxygen-carrying capacity you lose in increased resistance in the circulation of blood.

"After losing a pint of blood, the athlete cannot train properly. This impairs training when the athlete needs it most. My impression is that 'blood doping' is not worth the effort and ordeal."

Matti Hannus, a famous Finnish sports reporter, says: "There's a rumor that Lasse Viren won his gold medals by blood doping. I don't believe it. How is it possible that in April he ran 25 kilometers in 1:14:21, which is world record time? In May, he won the Finnish cross-country title? In June, he ran 10,000 meters in 27:43 and in July, he conquered the world at Montreal? Do you want to tell me that he had four blood transfusions?"

6.

What You Should Eat

Paul Anderson, who raised the greatest weight ever lifted by a human — 6,270 pounds — would use his bare hands to squeeze the blood from two pounds of raw hamburger into a glass of tomato juice and would then drink the mixture.

Wayne Stetina, a top U.S. distance bicycle racer, is a vegetarian and carries a twenty-pound Crockpot, apples, nuts, bulbs, and plants wherever he races. In the Olympic village, he grew lentil seeds in a huge plastic bag by the window. "His room is always full of shells, peels, and cores," a roommate complains.

Park Barner, the world record holder for the 100 kilometer run, fasts regularly before he races.

First baseman Ron Blumberg of the Chicago White Sox gorges on food. "Once the team went to a restaurant that serves an all-you-can-eat smorgasbord," a teammate reports. "The main courses consisted of shrimp, lobster, and steak, and Blumberg really loaded up. When the team was leaving the restaurant, the owner tore up his check and begged Blumberg not to return."

Kyle Rote, Jr., of the North American Soccer League and winner of three Superstars competitions, is a keen student of nutrition and relies on the scientifically sound diet his wife devised. His only idiosyncrasy is a fetish for bananas.

These stories prove a point: Whether you're a meat eater or a vegetarian, a faster or a gorger, you can be a standout in competitive sports.

"Eighteen Dozen Eggs a Week"

I had heard that Jim Montgomery (winner of four gold medals in the 1976 Olympics) had a fantastic appetite; that his mother buys eighteen dozen eggs a week. I could hardly believe it.

When he came for his recruitment trip, I decided to let him get his own breakfast and just put everything out. He ate eight eggs, a pound of bacon, a loaf of bread, and drank almost a quart of orange juice. And that was just breakfast! He really lived up to his advance billing. He is some eater.

— MARJORIE COUNSILMAN,
wife of Olympic swimming coach Doc Counsilman

Do Athletes Really Need Special Foods?

A multimillion-dollar industry has sprung up to supply an answer with "energy" and "body-building" foods, vitamins, minerals, and drugs. They are as exotic as anabolic steroids and as commonplace as protein supplements and sugared beverages.

In my opinion, none of them is needed, nor is there any need for a special training table. The body can be kept healthy with good basic foods — milk, eggs, meat, poultry, fish, fresh fruits and vegetables.

As long as ample nutrients of all kinds are obtained, quantity and variety for the most part should be the key ingredients in determining an exerciser's diet.

Early in my running career, I grasped for any competitive advantage. I consumed vitamin pills in large quantities, took wheat germ oil by the tablespoon, and popped bone meal tablets. I spent a few weeks avoiding starch, but I became so weak that I couldn't run. Once I became a vegetarian. But my children wouldn't put up with that and demanded meat on the family table. Another time I drank so much milk the cholesterol level in my blood became abnormally high.

Yet I was not as bad as some.

Here is a partial list of diet supplements I know athletes have taken: vitamins, iodine, magnesium, manganese, selenium, copper, zinc, calcium, potassium, sodium chloride, phosphorus, kelp, garlic, brewer's yeast, bee pollen, bone meal, lecithin, desiccated liver, ginseng, wheat germ, and pumpkin and sunflower seeds.

After years of experimenting on myself, I now know what nutritionists have known for decades: Everything your body needs can be supplied by a proper diet.

The same rules for eating apply universally to those who exercise and those who don't. The only difference is that people who are physically active require more calories and more fluids.

The Essential Nutrients

To remain healthy, your body requires more than forty nutrients, which are found in the six components of food — water, carbohydrates, fat, protein, minerals, and vitamins.

Water

You can safely omit the other nutrients for weeks or even months, but without water you can't survive for even a few days.

Even if you don't exercise, your body requires at least six glasses of fluid a day. (Some of the fluid requirement can be met in the food you eat.) When you exercise, you need far more fluid. Drink at least a glass of fluid with every meal and whenever you are thirsty. Don't wait for thirst to drink — by that time your body may have lost three to five glasses of fluid. If you have normal kidneys, don't worry about drinking too much fluid. Dr. Jack Crawford, professor of pediatrics at Harvard Medical School, has shown that healthy adults can tolerate up to eighty glasses of fluid for one day.

Water is the main component of cells, urine, sweat, and blood. When you are dehydrated, your cells become dehydrated and chemical reactions in the cells are impaired. The cells can't build tissue and can't utilize energy efficiently. You don't produce urine, and consequently toxic products build up in your bloodstream. You don't sweat, so your temperature rises. Your blood volume decreases and you have less blood to transport oxygen and nutrients through your body. The result is that your muscles become weak and you become tired.

You obtain water from almost anything you eat or drink. Water is also the by-product of every chemical reaction that produces energy in your body.

Carbohydrates

Carbohydrates are components of food that are composed of carbon, oxygen, and hydrogen (hence the name carb o hydrate). They are the primary source of energy during vigorous exercise. One or more basic sugar molecules bind together to form all carbohydrates.

In foods, sugar molecules may exist individually and are called monosaccharides; in pairs they're called disaccharides, or in chains of three or more, polysaccharides. Disaccharides and polysaccharides must be broken down into monosaccharides before they can be absorbed into the body.

Only three monosaccharides — glucose, fructose, and galactose — can pass from the intestine into the bloodstream and then to the liver. In the liver, fructose and galactose are converted into glucose so that glucose is the

> I took some of the best long-distance runners in America and I dehydrated them with diuretics. After they ran for 55 minutes, they all passed out.
> —DAVID L. COSTILL, Ph.D., *Director of the Human Performance Laboratory at Ball State University*

Athletes Fuel Up on Carbohydrates

Mary Decker, a world-class half miler at age fourteen, would insist on a plate of plain spaghetti three hours before a race. "At the time, everyone thought that she was strange," remarks Brooks Johnson, former U.S. Olympic track coach. "Now runners realize that spaghetti is loaded with carbohydrates."

Oliver Martin, coach of the U.S. Olympic distance cycling team, says, "It is amazing how much food — mostly carbohydrates — a European professional cyclist will consume on a long ride. I've seen riders eat ten sandwiches containing marmalade, jam and cheese. U.S. riders are finally realizing they must eat more. I would never go on a five-hour ride and drink only water. I would BONK out. My body would run out of fuel."

At one sitting Jim Montgomery and Ron Blumberg can consume a large loaf of bread apiece.

Kyle Rote's bananas are a good source of carbohydrates.

only circulating form of carbohydrate that is used for energy.

Table sugar and honey both contain glucose in a form that is so quickly absorbed that it goes into your bloodstream almost immediately. Starches require several steps to be broken down into monosaccharides and thus are absorbed more slowly. Potatoes, bread, spaghetti, and macaroni are sources of starch. Cellulose is a polysaccharide that is composed of such long chains of sugars that our bodies can't even break them down and they are excreted in our stools. Lettuce, whole grains, cabbage, and celery are sources of cellulose.

Fats

Fats are greasy to the touch and insoluble in water. They are the primary source of muscle energy at rest, and they provide energy late in endurance events after muscles have been depleted of much of their glycogen. Visible fats include margarine, butter, salad and cooking oils, bacon fat, and cream, and some of the fat on meat. Invisible fats are found in egg yolk, meats, olives, whole milk, avocados, and nuts. Fat yields 4,082 calories per pound, which is more than twice as much as carbohydrate.

Fat is classified as primarily saturated or primarily unsaturated. Saturated fats are usually found in animals, and when eaten in large amounts are thought to predispose to heart attacks. Unsaturated fats are usually found in plants, and although they were once thought to be helpful in preventing heart attacks, this is now subject to controversy.

Fat is stored in the body around the organs and in larger quantities under the skin in overweight people. Athletes store fat in their muscles.

Protein

Protein is an organic substance that is the primary structural material of cells and tissue. It is never a source of immediate energy and protein requirements do not increase with exercise. The body has no means to store extra protein. Proteins are found in milk, meats, eggs, cheeses, grains, and legumes.

Protein contains twenty-three different amino acids but the body can manufacture only fourteen of them. Thus every person must obtain nine amino acids from his daily diet. They are known as the essential amino acids.

Before protein is absorbed into the bloodstream, it is broken down into its basic building blocks, the amino acids. Thus the body is unable to recognize whether its source of protein comes from meat, fish, or peanuts.

Food sources of protein are classified as complete — containing all nine essential amino acids, and usually found in animal tissue — and incomplete — lacking one or more of the essential amino acids, and usually found in plant tissue. It is not necessary that you eat protein sources, such as meat, that contain all the essential amino acids. By combining corn, which has only seven of the essential amino acids, with beans, which have the two missing ones, you can satisfy all your protein requirements.

Minerals

Minerals are basic chemicals found in the soil. Plants pick up minerals from the soil. Animals obtain their minerals when they eat plants, and man obtains his minerals when he eats either plants or animals.

Minerals are essential to the conduction of nerve impulses and control heartbeat and the contraction of all muscles. They control the amount of water your body can hold and regulate how it is stored.

They are found in all plant and animal material. Fruits, vegetables, grains, and nuts are particularly rich sources of minerals. More information on minerals will be found in Chapter 8.

Vitamins

Vitamins are components of enzymes that regulate the rate that chemical reactions proceed in the body. They are not a direct source of energy and their requirements do not increase significantly during exercise. More information on vitamins will be found in Chapter 7.

Vitamins only act on nutrients. That's why taking massive amounts of vitamins will not protect you from a diet deficient in any of the other essential nutrients. Using vitamins in place of a meal makes no sense whatsoever.

Vitamins are found in almost any food you eat except sugar. Since different vitamins come from many different sources, you should vary your foods as much as possible.

The Four-Food Plan

Nobody knows the perfect combination of carbohydrates, fats, protein, vitamins, minerals, and liquids. How much zinc, vitamin C, calcium, and other nutrients your body needs is still debated. However, during World War II, the National Academy of Sciences established Recommended Daily Allowances (R.D.A.) for several of the body's main nutrients and now has established values for seventeen. These are the amounts of nutrients that you need to keep healthy.

It is not necessary to know the R.D.A. for each of the nutrients. To insure that you eat the right foods in the right amounts, simply follow the Four-Food Plan, a simple diet guide that was first published by the U.S. Department of Agriculture during World War II and improved in 1956. Each food has been assigned to one of four groups of foods similar in nutritional value. The system is based on the principle that it doesn't matter whether your vitamin C comes from a raisin, an apple, or a walnut, or your protein from meat, corn and beans, chicken, or fish. Your body breaks down all food, regardless of its source, into its basic elements before using it.

The beauty of the Four-Food Plan is its flexibility and simplicity. You don't have to have a Ph.D. in nutrition to get a balanced diet. If you follow the Four-Food Plan, all your nutritional needs will be fulfilled.

1. *Fruits and vegetables* Fruits and vegetables are an excellent and inexpensive source of minerals, vitamins, and carbohydrates. Because they contain more bulk and relatively fewer calories than the other groups, they are an excellent food for a weight-loss program.

2. *The cereal and grain group* Bread, cereal, flour, and baked goods are a rich source of carbohydrates, protein, and minerals. They also contain vitamins and a small amount of fat.

3. *The high protein group* This group includes meat, fish, poultry, eggs, legumes, and nuts.

Because of the saturated fat content of meats and eggs, which has been implicated in heart disease, I recommend that you limit your meat and egg consumption to four servings or less of each per week. You should obtain most of your protein requirements from chicken, fish, legumes,

A Four-Food Plan Diet under 2,000 Calories

	GROUP 1 FRUITS AND VEGETABLES	GROUP 2 CEREALS AND GRAINS	GROUP 3 MEAT AND HIGH-PROTEIN FOOD	GROUP 4 MILK AND OTHER DAIRY PRODUCTS
BREAKFAST	orange juice, 1 glass — 100 calories	cooked oatmeal, sm. bowl, 1 tsp. sugar — 120 calories; toast, 2 slices — 120 calories		milk, 1 glass — 150 calories butter, 1 tablespoon — 50 calories
LUNCH	apple — 75 calories lettuce — 15 calories	bread for sandwich — 120 calories		cheese for sandwich, 2 slices — 75 calories milk, 1 glass — 150 calories
DINNER	lettuce and tomato salad — 75 calories potato — 120 calories strawberries, 1 cup — 60 calories	corn-on-cob — 100 calories	salmon, 4 oz. — 200 calories; green beans, sm. serving — 75 calories	butter, 1 tablespoon — 50 calories
SNACK	banana — 130 calories		peanuts, ¼ cup — 200 calories	
NUMBER OF SERVINGS	7	4	3	5

and nuts. Legumes are a neglected source of protein. The legume family includes navy beans, kidney beans, lima beans, stringbeans, soy beans, lentils, black-eyed peas, peas, and peanuts.

4. *Milk and milk products group* Milk and cheese provide a rich source of protein, calcium, and riboflavin. You should limit your intake of whole milk because of its high fat content. If you drink a lot of milk, drink low-fat or skim milk or buttermilk.

If you consume four large servings of the first two groups (fruits and vegetables, cereals and grains) and two large servings of the last two groups (high protein, milk and milk products) each day, you will supply your nutritional needs for carbohydrates, fats, proteins, vitamins, and minerals. If you need more fluid, drink any fluid you prefer. If you need more calories, eat more of the foods of your choice.

A Balanced Diet for Vegetarians

What about vegetarians? They can have a balanced diet by following a six-food plan recommended by nutritionists:

1. Fruit
2. Vegetables
3. Milk, dairy and poultry products, including eggs
4. Bread and cereal
5. Legumes
6. Nuts

At least three servings of each of the first four groups and one serving of each of the last two each day will furnish the vegetarian's nutritional needs.

Vegetarian Athletes

Maurice Lucas, Bill Walton, and Jack Ramsay of the Portland Trailblazers basketball team
Michael "Campy" Russell, Jim Brewer, Austin Carr of the Cleveland Cavaliers basketball team
Connie Hawkins of the Atlanta Hawks
Siegfried Bauer, who ran the length of New Zealand — 1,350 miles — in eighteen days

The 3,000-Calorie Vegetarian Diet

	calories	calories
BREAKFAST		600
8-oz. glass of fruit juice	100	
(grapefruit 80, orange 100, apple 120)		
bowl of unsweetened whole grain or bran cereal, with wheat germ, sesame seeds, or dried fruit, with apple juice	200	
peanut butter or avocado sandwich on whole wheat bread	300	
LUNCHEON		900
mixed raw vegetables (celery, carrots, cauliflower)	100	
2 slices of whole wheat bread with tahini and hummus or equivalent bean, nut, and seed paste with oil, lemon juice, and seasoning	500	
8-oz. bowl of vegetable soup or glass of vegetable juice	100	
2 fresh fruits	200	
(apple 75, orange 90, grapefruit 100, banana 130)		
DINNER		1,500
tossed salad with one avocado and oil and lemon dressing and a glass of vegetable juice	400	
8-oz. serving of nut roast, lentils and brown rice, or stuffed squash	250	
8-oz. serving of beans, corn, spaghetti, or sweet potatoes	200	
8-oz. serving of steamed green, leafy vegetables such as turnip greens, mustard greens, collards, broccoli	100	
slice of fruit pie or 4-oz. serving of dried fruit	350	
		3,000

This basic 3,000-calorie diet can be expanded readily to 4,000 or more calories by increasing the size of the portions, snacking on 4 ounces of nuts and seeds, or 8 ounces of dried fruit (500 calories), or by adding moderate amounts of yellow cheeses (100 calories/ounce), eggs (100 calories), and beer or wine (150 calories/glass).

SOURCE: Alex Hershaft, Ph.D., President, Vegetarian Information Service, P.O. Box 5888, Washington, D.C. 20014

The complete vegetarian who abstains from all animal products — including eggs and milk — can simply eliminate Group 3 and increase Group 5 to at least four servings a day. However, special provision needs to be made for obtaining vitamin B_{12}.

Limit Fat, Sugar, and Salt Intake

The average American eats too much red meat, salt, and sugar. While exercise may offer some degree of protection from the ravages of dietary indiscretions, I *strongly* recommend that you limit your intake of these foodstuffs. Many other physicians and nutritionists urge that we change our way of eating. A recent U.S. Senate committee report went so far as to recommend that every family reduce consumption of salt, refined sugar, and fat. It urges us to eat more fruits, vegetables, whole grains, poultry, fish, and skim milk.

Fat

Fat makes food taste good. Without it, you probably wouldn't enjoy eating. But the ingestion of excessive amounts of saturated fat is associated with heart disease and strokes, and the amount of saturated fat in the average American's diet should be sharply reduced.

Saturated fat Saturated fats are usually of animal origin — the fats in meat, whole milk, cream, butter, cheese, and lard. Some saturated fats are of vegetable origin: coconut oil (very highly saturated), solid margarines, and hydrogenated vegetable oil. A good rule-of-thumb is that you can assume a fat is saturated if it comes in solid form.

Saturated fats have the effect of raising the cholesterol level, a type of fat in the blood, and many studies have associated a high level of serum cholesterol with a high incidence of heart disease. The level of cholesterol in the blood is one way of predicting your chances of having a heart attack: people who have cholesterol levels of over 260 mg./100 cc. have more than twice the chance of developing heart disease than those at lower levels. You can have any physician order this test on you.

Dietary Goals for the United States Prepared by the Select Committee on Nutrition and Human Needs of the United States Senate February 1977

RECOMMENDED GOALS

1. Increase carbohydrate consumption to account for 55 to 60 percent of the energy (caloric) intake.

2. Reduce overall fat consumption from approximately 40 to 30 percent of energy intake.

3. Reduce saturated fat consumption to account for about 10 percent of total energy intake; and balance that with polyunsaturated and monounsaturated fats, which should account for about 10 percent of energy intake each.

4. Reduce cholesterol consumption to about 300 mg. a day.

5. Reduce sugar consumption by about 40 percent to account for about 15 percent of total energy intake.

6. Reduce salt consumption by about 50 to 85 percent to approximately 3 grams a day.

THE GOALS SUGGEST THE FOLLOWING CHANGES IN FOOD SELECTION AND PREPARATION

1. Increase consumption of fruits and vegetables and whole grains.

2. Decrease consumption of meat and increase consumption of poultry and fish.

3. Decrease consumption of foods high in fat and partially substitute polyunsaturated fat for saturated fat.

4. Substitute non-fat milk for whole milk.

5. Decrease consumption of butterfat, eggs and other high cholesterol sources.

6. Decrease consumption of sugar and foods high in sugar content.

7. Decrease consumption of salt and foods high in salt content.

Approximate Composition of Common Food Fats

	CHOLESTEROL (MILLIGRAMS)	% POLY-UNSATURATES	% MONO-UNSATURATES	% SATURATES
OILS:				
Coconut	0	0	8	92
Cocoa Butter	0	5	34	61
Corn	0	58	31	11
Cottonseed	0	59	16	25
Olive	0	7	81	12
Peanut	0	31	46	23
Safflower	0	78	12	10
Sesame	0	43	43	14
Soybean	0	63	21	16
Sunflower	0	53	15	12
FATS:				
Butter (1 tablespoon)	30	4	37	59
Lard (1 tablespoon)	13	10	52	38
Crisco	0	26	49	25
Regular hydrogenated shortening	0	7	70	23

	% CHOLESTEROL	% POLY-UNSATURATES	% SATURATES
MARGARINE:			
Fleischmann's (stick)	0	27	20
Mazola (stick)	0	30	22
Promise (stick)	0	48	17
Fleischmann's (tub)	0	36	20
Mazola (tub)	0	37	23
Promise (tub)	0	63	15

SOURCE: From *Live High on Low Fat*. Copyright © 1962 by Sylvia Rosenthal. Reprinted by permission of J.B. Lippincott Company.

Cholesterol Cholesterol is manufactured by the body and is necessary to it for many reasons: to insulate nerves, to serve as a building material for the sex hormones, to carry fat through the body, and to help defend against infection. However, excess cholesterol in the bloodstream collects on the inner walls of blood vessels and forms plaques. As the plaques enlarge with the continuing deposits of cholesterol,

Golfer Gary Player, a longtime advocate of physical fitness and a recent winner of three consecutive Professional Golfers Association tournaments at the unprecedented age of forty-two, avoids sugar, white flour, meat, coffee, and ordinary (nonherbal) tea.

Americans Eat Too Much Fat

	AVERAGE AMERICAN DIET	RECOMMENDED DIET
Carbohydrates	40%	60%
Fat	40%	25%
Protein	20%	15%

Cholesterol Content of Some Foods

FOOD*	AMOUNT†	CHOLESTEROL (MILLIGRAMS)
Brains	2 ounces	1,700
Butter fat	3½ ounces	280
Buttermilk (skim)	1 cup	5
Cheese (Cheddar)	1 ounce	27
Cheese (Mozzarella, partially skim)	1 ounce	18
Cheese (Parmesan)	1 tablespoon	5
Cream, heavy	1 tablespoon	20
Crab meat	3½ ounces	161
Clams	3½ ounces	114
Egg yolk	1	250
Fish	3½ ounces	70
Ice cream	1 cup	53
Ice milk	1 cup	26
Kidney	2 ounces	250
Liver	3½ ounces	300
Lobster	3½ ounces	85
Meat (lean)	3½ ounces	94
Milk, skim	1 cup	7
Milk, whole	1 cup	30
Oysters	3½ ounces	200
Poultry	3½ ounces	75
Scallops	3½ ounces	53
Shrimps	3½ ounces	150
Sweetbreads	3 ounces	396
Veal	3½ ounces	90
Yogurt (low-fat)	8-ounce carton	17

(Figures from U.S. Department of Agriculture *Composition of Food* and American Medical Association, Department of Foods and Nutrition)

*Meats, poultry, and fish are cooked weight.
†3½ ounces are approximately 100 grams.

SOURCE: From *Live High on Low Fat.* Copyright © 1962 by Sylvia Rosenthal. Reprinted by permission of J.B. Lippincott Company.

the arteries become clogged or may fill up entirely, resulting in arteriosclerosis (hardening of the arteries), angina, and heart attack or stroke.

Other animals also manufacture cholesterol, and it is thought that consuming foods high in cholesterol will increase the level of cholesterol in your own bloodstream. Foods especially high in cholesterol are brains, organ meats, and egg yolks (high in both saturated fat and cholesterol).

Other fats There are two other types of fat: monounsaturated and polyunsaturated. Neither of these fats have the effect of raising the serum cholesterol level, and indeed polyunsaturated fats were formerly believed to tend to lower the level of cholesterol in the blood, but now this point is controversial. Olive oil is an example of a monounsaturated fat. Polyunsaturated fats, which are usually liquid oils of vegetable origin, include corn, cottonseed, and safflower oil.

Sugar

Each year the average American eats his or her weight in sugar, and the per capita consumption of sugar increases year by year. The American sweet tooth is reflected not only in the abundance of sugary foods such as candy, cake, jams, sugarcoated cereals, and soft drinks, but also in the fact that it is an invisible ingredient in such items as bread, canned soups and sauces, and many other processed foods. If you don't believe me, read the labels on some products the next time you go marketing. Some people substitute honey, brown sugar, or molasses under the impression that they are thereby avoiding the ill effects of eating refined sugar. They are mistaken. These are all just another form of sugar.

Aside from the fact that sugar causes tooth decay, your intake of sugar should be sharply limited for the following reasons:

Sugar makes you hungry. When you eat sugar, your blood sugar level rises and your body responds by producing a hormone called insulin. This hormone causes a rapid drop of your blood sugar level, and within a few hours, your blood sugar level drops and you get hungry. This is called rebound hypoglycemia.

Sugar has little nutritional value. Sugar contains only calories. When you exercise, your body requires increased amounts of minerals and other nutrients, and sugar contains none of these.

Sugar may cause heart attacks. Cholesterol may not be the only culprit. Several studies show that patients who have

My 4,325-Calorie Training Diet with Limited Amounts of Salt, Sugar, and Fat

BREAKFAST	*calories*
orange juice, 2 glasses	200
oatmeal, 4 cups	600
raisins, ½ cup	250
toast, 2 pieces	120
butter, 1 tablespoon	50

LUNCH	
cream cheese sandwich with lettuce and tomato	200
tuna sandwich	300
apple juice, 1 glass	120
orange, 1 medium	90

SNACK	
orange, 1 medium	90
banana, 1 medium	130

DINNER	
chicken, 1 breast	210
chicken, 1 leg	200
potato	120
bread, 8 pieces	480
butter, 3 tablespoons	150
leafy green vegetable salad with vinegar and oil	300
corn-on-the-cob	100
pear, 1 medium	75

SNACK	
peanut butter sandwich	175
cashews, ¼ pound	200
orange, 1 medium	90
plum, 1	75
Total:	4,325

SOURCE: Gabe Mirkin, M.D.

suffered from heart attacks have a sweet tooth. Before their heart attacks, they ate far more sugar than the general population.

Dr. John Yudkin, professor of nutrition at the University of London in England, is the leading expert on the dietary sugar–heart attack link. He demonstrated that increasing the amount of sugar in the diet raises fat levels in the blood.

Dr. George Mann, a professor of nutrition at Vanderbilt University Medical School in Tennessee, demonstrated that decreasing the amount of sugar in the diet lowers the fat levels in the blood.

All societies that have a high sugar intake have a high incidence of heart attacks. But not all societies that have a high cholesterol intake have an increased incidence of heart attacks. The Samburu and Masai in East Africa and the tribesmen in Mongolia eat tremendous amounts of animal fat. But they eat no refined sugar and rarely suffer from heart attacks.

Salt

Even though you need only one-fifth of a gram of salt a day, the average American eats between six and eighteen grams.

A high salt diet is associated with high blood pressure which, in turn, is associated with heart attacks and strokes. There is also some evidence that taking excess salt in your diet may limit your ability to exercise in hot weather. For a fuller discussion of salt see Chapter 8.

How Many Calories Do You Need?

If you exercise frequently or compete in sports, expect to consume more food than the average person. You need the food to supply energy for your muscles.

A study of the Australian Olympic team showed that more than 30 percent of its members devoured more than 4,000 calories a day. The average American consumes about 3,000 calories.

In training camp, some members of the Boston Celtics eat 8,000 to 10,000 calories a day. Even on that huge intake — three times the amount of the average male — most players lose weight. Guard Charlie Scott once lost twelve pounds in ten days.

Long-distance cyclists can burn up to 10,000 calories in riding as many as a hundred and fifty miles a day. For a vegetarian like Wayne Stetina, getting a massive amount of calories can be a problem. In Olympic village he was known as an all-night muncher.

Whenever I lecture about the tremendous calorie requirements of modern-day athletes, people in the audience often ask about the Tarahumaras in Mexico. In spite of a meager diet of only 1,500 calories per day, they are able to participate in a religious ceremony that involves kicking a ball more than two hundred continuous miles. Their feats of endurance are legendary.

But they couldn't possibly compete against modern athletes. Their meager diets wouldn't give them enough fuel to perform the tremendous workloads that athletes use in training today.

Exercise and Obesity

Hard exercise usually protects you from obesity. Food passes through your system faster, decreasing the absorption of calories. You're not as hungry, and you even burn more calories after you exercise.

When I'm hobbled by an injury or succumb to inertia — meaning that I don't run five to ten miles a day — I'm starving and eat all the time. I gain weight. As long as I run frequently, I remain lean.

An athlete should cut back on eating after his competitive days are over. It is the extra food which is not converted to energy, and not muscles turning to fat, that causes some former athletes to become obese.

Several studies have shown that people who were athletes in their youth and became sedentary in adult life are more susceptible to heart attacks than people who have never exercised at all. While scientists don't agree on the cause, I suspect that these people adopted poor eating habits early in life. They ate too much and what they did eat contained too much fat, salt, and sugar. As long as they were active, they avoided obesity. But as time passed, they became less active and continued their dietary indiscretions, which made them more susceptible to heart attacks.

When I first met Gabe Mirkin, I was impressed by his slim figure. I thought he had to be watching every calorie to remain that thin. I was astounded when I saw what he normally ate for lunch, dinner, and snacks. He had to be consuming at least one-and-a-half to two times the calories I was and yet he was 15 pounds lighter. He is 6 feet tall and weighs 140 pounds.

Gabe has learned the secret of remaining slim — burn off excessive calories with exercise.

— RONALD SHORE, M.D.

Body Fat

Many athletes who appear to be fat really are not. Vasili Alexeev, the Russian weight lifter who holds more than seventy-five world records, has extraordinary muscles. They are so large that they look like fat. Yet he has less than 12 percent body fat, compared to 15 percent for the average American male and 25 percent for the average female.

Many 300-pound football players have far less fat than the average person. Dr. Ancel Keys of the University of Minnesota calls these athletes "overweight, but underfat."

The highest percentage of body fat we could find in the National Football League was 22 percent and that was on a 240-pound tackle. A New York Jets halfback who weighed in at 195 pounds had almost zero percent body fat — the same as that of gymnasts Stephanie Willim and Olga Korbut. The lowest percentage recorded in a marathon runner was Gary Tuttle's 1.4 percent.

You can easily identify a fitness buff or athlete in a crowd. They have very little body fat. An athlete stores fat in his or her muscles; muscle fat is not visible. It doesn't even make muscles bulge. Nonathletes store fat under the skin. In gives them unsightly bulges around the waist, buttocks, thighs, hips, and breasts.

A body caliper, which looks like an engineer's compass, can be used to measure your percentage of body fat. Calipers are used in many fitness and weight reduction programs and can be bought for about $100 at stores that sell fitness equipment.

A caliper works on the principle that fat is stored under the skin. The more fat you have in your body, the thicker the layer of fat under your skin. The caliper is used to measure the thickness of your skin. From tables, you can then read off your percentage of body fat.

A more sophisticated means of measuring body fat is based on the principle that fat is less dense than muscle. The fatter you are, the more water you displace. That's why fat people float better than muscular people. The volume of water displaced by your body can be used to compute your percentage of body fat. The water displacement method is far more complex and time consuming; it can take from forty-five to sixty minutes.

Jack Mahurin, a professor of exercise physiology at Springfield College, uses the caliper method when he tests large numbers of people. "Even though a caliper method is less accurate, I can measure fifty people with it in the same time it takes to measure one with the water displacement method."

One Meal a Day or Many?

It has been shown scientifically that the body uses calories more efficiently if they are taken in multiple small meals. A single large meal overloads the body system and the excess calories are stored as fat in the blood and tissue.

The average American drinks coffee for breakfast, downs a sandwich for lunch, and devours thousands of calories in the evening. It is the big evening intake of calories that makes Americans obese and prone to heart attacks.

Clarence Cohn, formerly of Michael Reese Hospital in Chicago, Illinois, studied two groups of rats. Both ate the same number of calories, but one group nibbled throughout the day and the other ate all their food in one meal. The nibblers had lower blood fat levels and lived longer.

Drs. Howard W. Haggard and Leon A. Greenberg found that workers performed better on five meals a day than on two. Waid W. Tuttle, in 1951, showed that workers who skipped breakfast performed less efficiently. J. Causeret, a French physician, studied Moslem distance runners in South Africa. During the Ramadan period, Moslems eat twice a day — before daybreak and at sunset. At other times they eat three meals a day. The runners performed better on three meals than on two.

The Great Protein Myth

Twenty years ago, Jean Mayer, a former Harvard nutritionist who is now the president of Tufts University and a syndicated newspaper columnist, taught his classes about the value of carbohydrates as a fuel for muscular exercise. At the very same time, Harvard's coaches took us out for steak dinners before competition, and meat was frequently served at the Varsity Club. The academic department was preaching carbohydrates while the athletic department was promoting proteins.

The great protein myth still exists today. Some sellers of protein supplements say that their product supplies quick energy and builds stronger muscles.

Six Meals a Day

Steve Pecher, the North American Soccer League's Rookie of the Year, eats at least six meals a day.

"He is the reason we eat cheeseburgers after a game," says teammate Kyle Rote, Jr. "He's got such a craving for them. It is nothing for him to eat three cheeseburgers with a full load of french fries and salad.

"On the day of a road trip, he'll have breakfast at home. On the way to the airport, he'll stop at a McDonald's to get an Egg McMuffin. While the team is waiting for the plane, he'll snack on French pastry. He'll eat the lunch served on the plane and have another lunch at the hotel. At 4 P.M. he will eat the pre-game meal.

"It is either his metabolism or the fact that we play or work out every day."

Rote is a five-meal-a-day athlete, but he eats smaller portions.

As early as 1866, two German physiologists, Voit and Pettenkofen, wrote a classic paper that showed that protein is not an immediate source of muscular energy. Their work has been repeatedly confirmed in the scientific literature. The Federal Trade Commission report says: "The scientific community is unequivocal and undivided in its rejection of the claim that protein provided quick energy."

Because muscle is composed of protein, some athletes, coaches, and trainers believe that protein supplements make muscles stronger. The only time that protein supplements can help build stronger muscles is when the athlete is not eating enough protein in his diet. Inadequate protein intake is almost never a problem for American athletes.

Scientists have shown that even with heavy exercise protein requirements do not rise significantly. In 1902, Dr. Russell Chittenden of Yale demonstrated that athletes can train and win international championships while eating a low-protein diet. Many other scientific studies since then have confirmed that a protein-rich diet does not improve performance. Dr. Frank Consolazio, who has done extensive testing on protein in the diet, says: "The additional protein doesn't enhance work performance."

His views are supported by many other studies. Unlike carbohydrates and fat, protein cannot be stored in the body. When presented to the body it must be used immediately or it is broken down by the liver and excreted through the kidneys in the urine. If you take more protein than your body can use, you force your liver and kidneys to work harder.

Athletes eat so much protein in their diet that the protein derived from supplements becomes insignificant. Dr. Autti Ahlstrom of the Universtiy of Tampere, Finland, analyzed the diets of several leading athletes who took protein supplements. He found that the supplements contributed less than 3 percent to their total protein intake.

Despite all the evidence, a $70-million-a-year protein supplement business has aimed much of its advertising at the athlete.

Many athletes still eat steak before competition.

"I'm as carnivorous as hell," exclaims Buddy Baker, a top NASCAR driver. "I eat a breakfast steak, tea with lemon and sugar before a race."

Other regular steak eaters: Derek Sanderson and Bobby Orr (hockey), Muhammad Ali, Emil Griffith, and Jerry Quarry (boxing), Stephanie Willim (gymnastics), and Dan Gable (wrestling).

Most of the pro football and hockey teams offer steak on the pre-game training table. Butch Buchholz eats a cheeseburger patty or eggs some two to three hours before his tennis matches. Both are loaded with protein.

Oliver Martin says, "Ninety-nine percent of all distance cyclers are steak-and-potato men." Gil Clancy, trainer of many famous boxing champions, swears by the high-protein diet. The strongest supporters of a high-protein diet are weight lifters.

The Russian weight lifters bring their own food to meets, including lots of caviar. "That's their protein supplement," says a top U.S. weight lifter. "It's almost pure protein, top prime stuff too."

Eating before Competing

You should enter a competition with an empty stomach. If you have food in your stomach, you will probably develop stomach cramps. Here's why: To aid digestion, the heart pumps a large volume of blood to the stomach. During exercise, the heart pumps blood to the muscles and the flow of blood to the stomach is greatly diminished. Without the blood supply, the stomach muscles suffer from lack of oxygen — and, like any muscle without oxygen, develop cramps.

The time it takes for the stomach to empty varies among individuals and can even vary in the same person from one time to another. Several factors determine how quickly your stomach empties — your level of conditioning, your emotional status, and what you eat.

Level of conditioning

When I first started to train, I had to eat at least six hours before a training session, but as my level of conditioning improved, what and when I ate was not as important. Sometimes I would eat a sandwich before an easy workout. The explanation: When your heart is in poor shape, it can't pump enough blood to supply your muscles and stomach at the same time. But as you become more fit, your heart becomes strong enough to supply both systems at the same time, provided that you are not exercising at full tilt. When I competed, I allowed three hours for my stomach to empty.

Emotional status

Using an X ray, Dr. Donald Cooper of Oklahoma State University studied how quickly food passes through the stomach. He found that football players required two to four hours longer for their stomachs to empty on game days than on nongame days, presumably because of stress.

What the athlete believes to be the best pre-competition meal may be more important than the meal itself. As Kyle Rote, Jr., says, "Science has gone in cycles. First it's steak. Then it's carbohydrates. No one really knows and half of it is psychological anyway."

Jeff Fair, trainer at Oklahoma State University, studied the effects of different meals eaten before a two-mile run. He found no difference in his study and concluded that psychological factors are more important than the meal itself.

When Athletes Eat before a Game

O. J. Simpson doesn't eat on game days. Neither does Joe Namath.

Bill Russell, the former Boston Celtic superstar, had to eat at least eight hours before he played; otherwise he would chuck it all up.

Muhammad Ali prefers to eat six hours before a fight.

Gil Clancy has his fighters eat at 2:30 P.M. for a 10:00 P.M. fight.

The Baltimore Orioles eat four and a half hours before games.

Hockey players eat a full meal six hours before game time. Three hours before faceoff, many players take tea and honey.

Dan Gable eats four and a half hours before a wrestling match.

Swimmers coached by Doc Counsilman eat about three hours before a meet.

The New York Jets serve a pregame meal five hours before kickoff.

The Pre-game Meal

Medically, the pre-game meal should satisfy the following requirements:

Be high in carbohydrates, but low in sugar
Be low in protein and fat
Contain at least three glasses of liquid
Ward off hunger pains during competition
Be easily digestible

I recommend a glass of orange juice, cereal with low-fat milk, lightly buttered toast, potatoes, and a minimum of two more glasses of fluids at least three hours before competition.

A pre-game meal should be high in carbohydrates

Carbohydrates are athletic fuel. They rank as the best source of immediate energy for competition.

Foods high in carbohydrates are bread, spaghetti, macaroni, potatoes, porridge, fruit, and fruit juices.

Italian Nicola Pietrangeli, who holds the record for most Davis Cup appearances (164) was criticized unjustly for downing wine and spaghetti before matches. Both foods are rich in carbohydrates.

Wayne Stetina, an Olympic cyclist and a vegetarian, loads up on breads and vegetables. The pre-game meal for a cyclist extends into competition. He must continue to eat throughout the race. During long cycle races, which may last six days, cyclists eat small sandwiches, porridge, and fruit to supply energy.

Many pro football teams offer a carbohydrate meal. For example, the New York Jets serve toast, pancakes, salad, and fruit juice as part of their pre-game meal.

A pre-game meal must be low in sugar

Because sugar is pure carbohydrate — the quickest source of energy — it should be an ideal pre-competition meal. But it has one major drawback.

In most people, a meal loaded with sugar causes hunger pains two to five hours after it is consumed. This is because sugar enters the bloodstream very rapidly in the form of glucose, triggering the release of a high level of insulin to clear the blood of sugar. The result is low blood sugar, a

What Athletes Eat before Competition

On fight day, Muhammad Ali eats "one of those juicy Kosher steaks, well done, with all sorts of vegetables."

Eric Ostbye, a Swede who ranks as the world's best marathon runner over fifty years of age, fasts regularly before each race.

Weight lifter Mark Cameron says, "Before competition something high in carbohydrates — grapes and bananas — are the best."

In spite of all we know about the pre-competition meal, athletes still perform well on their own favorite foods.

Mike Torrez of the Boston Red Sox will not eat the same meal he consumed before pitching a losing game, only the meal he ate before his last winning effort.

Pro bowler Carmen Salvino eats anything. But "Jim Stefanich, one of my chief competitors, eats what I eat," says Salvino.

Derek Sanderson, sometimes considered a maverick in the National Hockey League, explains his feelings about the pre-game meal.

"As a kid, I didn't know anything and ate cheeseburgers and french fries. In the junior leagues, I learned about the value of a carbohydrate meal and ate carbohydrates. In the National Hockey League I eat steak and potatoes because I like them. I even smoke a pack of cigarettes before game time."

condition called "rebound hypoglycemia." Instead of sugar, eat fruit, which contains fructose. Because fructose has to be broken down in the liver into glucose before it can be used by the body, it passes into the bloodstream more slowly and is less likely to cause rebound hypoglycemia.

A large amount of sugar also draws water into the stomach and intestinal tract. This distends the stomach and often causes stomach cramps.

Honey, corn syrup, maple syrup, and molasses are almost 100 percent sugar and have the same drawbacks as sugar. However, a teaspoon or so of any form of sugar is usually not enough to create a problem.

A pre-game meal should be low in protein

Protein is never a source of immediate energy, so you don't need it in the pre-game meal.

Other drawbacks: The breakdown products of protein are similar to those of exercise and can cause fatigue. Because they can only be eliminated by the kidneys, they increase urination. However, if protein-laden food is eaten more than four hours before competition, these side effects are diminished.

A pre-game meal should be low in fat

Babe Ruth, the home-run king, once ate twenty hot dogs, which are full of fat, just before a game. His record stood until 1932, when two-ton Tony Galento broke Ruth's record by gorging on fifty-two wieners before a fight. Galento won that fight, but he never repeated his record-breaking eating performance.

These great athletes are the exception, not the rule. Remember: You won't be able to perform at your best after a fatty meal.

Pre-competition meals should contain at least three glasses of liquid

When you exercise, even at low-level intensity, you lose fluid. Besides sweating, you blow off water with each breath. When you lose 3 percent of your body weight in fluid, your temperature rises and your muscles heat up and have trouble contracting efficiently.

Once exercise begins, your body cannot absorb as much fluid as it loses. To get the most out of your performance, always start with extra fluid in your system. The one

Fluid Loss in Athletes

Phil Esposito of the New York Rangers can lose twelve pounds in a game. Paul Silas, formerly of the Boston Celtics, can lose seventeen pounds a game. Frank Shorter, the Olympic gold and silver medal winner in the marathon, has lost eight pounds in a race.

Even though they exercise in a fluid medium, swimmers lose fluid, Doc Counsilman says. Olympic medalist John Kinsella can lose three pounds in a workout.

drawback of drinking too much fluid: You'll have to urinate.

A pre-competition meal should be easily digestible

Several years ago, I coached a girls' track team in Baltimore. I recommended pancakes for a pre-race meal because of their high carbohydrate content.

Some of the girls ran their best times while others deposited their pancakes all along the cross-country course. Because pancakes are high in carbohydrates they should be an ideal pre-competition food. But not if they are loaded with butter (a source of fat) and syrup (a source of sugar).

Liquid meals

Dr. Donald Cooper tried to find a pre-game meal that would pass through the stomach quickly and still be nutritious. He settled on liquid meals that contained carbohydrates, fat, and protein and found that most players could eat these meals two and one half hours before game time and still have empty stomachs when they started to play.

"The players' impressions were so favorable that we are continuing to use the liquid meals and have begun to use them in other sports as well," writes Dr. Cooper.

Doc Counsilman uses liquid meals "when a swimmer has a preliminary race close to the finals or I have an athlete with a nervous stomach." But he says his athletes prefer a solid meal if they have time. "It seems to give them more satisfaction."

Liquid meals are commercially available and cost about $1.50 per serving.

Members of the University of Nebraska football team drink a high-energy liquid meal two and a half hours before each game in addition to their regular heavy meals.

What Athletes Prefer after Competition

After competition athletes need minerals and carbohydrates. That means beer for many.

"After playing in the hot weather, an athlete must replace his fuel," says soccer star Kyle Rote, Jr. "That's why most of the guys drink beer after a game."

Rote doesn't drink beer himself. He says he thinks "it destroys the brain cells."

Hockey player Derek Sanderson may drink "ten cold ones after a game." Baseball player Ron LeFlore drinks five. Every home team in the National Basketball Association serves a case of beer or soft drinks after a game. Football players follow each game with beer.

"Almost every tennis player in the world, both male and female, drinks beer after a game," says Butch Buchholz, the commissioner for World Team Tennis. "The alcohol goes out in the urine and the athlete can play the next day with no side effects."

7.

Vitamins

Massive Vitamin Dosage

Vitamins are part of enzymes that regulate chemical reactions in the body. They are necessary in small amounts for normal growth and maintenance of life. Because the body can't manufacture vitamins, it must obtain them from food or supplements.

Vitamin-popping is a national craze and the most notorious vitamin pill-takers are athletes. Pill-poppers feel that if vitamins keep them healthy, massive doses will make them super healthy. It's true that vitamins are essential to good health, but amounts in excess of what the body needs do no good and usually end up in the urine.

According to most medical experts, large amounts of vitamin supplements don't beef up performance, don't improve strength or endurance, and don't prevent injuries or colds. They are not even a source of energy. On the other hand, taking overdoses of vitamins can be dangerous.

A hazard of taking large doses of vitamin supplements is pointed out by Brooks Johnson, a track and field coach for the 1976 U.S. Olympic team: "If you are going to give athletes large amounts of supplements, you better make sure that they are still taking them at the time of their most important meets or competition. I am confident that the body develops a dependency for them."

Johnson, who recommends vitamins to his athletes, argues that "there are no scientific studies that spell out the vitamin requirements for a competitive athlete." He is right.

Many Athletes Take Vitamin Pills

One member of the U.S. Olympic cycling team has been reported to gobble vitamins by the handful. "He might take thirty a day," says a teammate.

Bob Scharf, an outstanding marathon runner in the 1960s, tops all pill-poppers that we interviewed. His daily dose: 51 pills. "If the pills work, I'll be a better athlete," he says. "If they don't, I'll only be wasting my money."

Although most of the professional trainers and coaches we interviewed felt that vitamin pills were of questionable value, they still made them available to all their athletes. Don Seeger, trainer of the Philadelphia Phillies, told us: "Some players feel they need vitamin pills. They see other teams taking them. If we didn't give it to them, they might go on strike. Personally, I don't believe in vitamins. I don't take them."

Virtually all the trainers believe that vitamin-taking is a personal decision. "We do not ask them to take vitamins, we just make them available," explains Tim Davey, a trainer for the New York Jets. "But eighty percent of the players use them."

While some teams offer only a simple one-a-day multivitamin, others serve up combinations of vitamins, minerals, protein, and bone meal tablets. "We've almost got a vitamin factory here," said one National Football League coach.

Bob Scharf's Daily Pills

Garlic	3
Lecithin	3
Zinc	3
Kelp	1
Desiccated liver	6
Bone meal	4
Multiple vitamin	4
Vitamin C, 500 milligrams	2
Vitamin E, 400 international units	2
Brewer's yeast	8
Wheat germ oil, 1 tablespoon	2
Pumpkin seeds, 1 tablespoon	1
Sunflower seeds, 1 tablespoon	1
Biotin	1
Bee pollen	3
Phosphate electrolytes	3
Ginseng	1
Chelated iron	1
B complex vitamins	2
Total Pills	51

Daily Vitamin Requirements

VITAMIN	SOURCE	RECOMMENDED DAILY ALLOWANCE
A	all yellow vegetables and fruits	5,000 units
B₁ (thiamine)	whole wheat and almost all plant and animal tissue	2 mgm.
B₂ (riboflavin)	milk and organ meat (liver, kidney, and brain)	2 mgm.
Niacinamide	yeast, meat, liver and poultry	20 mgm.
B₆ (pyridoxine)	wheat, bran, yeast, seeds, and corn	3 mgm.
Biotin	liver, yeast, egg yolk, tomato	.3 mgm.
Panthothenic acid	beef, yeast, egg yolk	15 mgm.
Folic acid	liver, green vegetables, cauliflower	.4 mgm.
B₁₂ (cyanoco-balamine)	all animal products	6 mgm.
C (ascorbic acid)	fruits	60 mgm.
D (calciferol)	vitamin D fortified milk	400 units
E (tocopherol)	milk, eggs, muscle meats, fish, cereals, leafy green vegetables, vegetable oil	30 units
K (menadione)	leafy green vegetables	2 mgm.

SOURCE: Gabe Mirkin, M.D., based on figures from the National Academy of Sciences

We found that as an athlete matures, he gets off the vitamin kick. Bobby Clarke and Muhammad Ali are prime examples. Bobby Clarke used to take 1,000 milligrams of vitamin C a day. He doesn't anymore.

"Dick Gregory, the comedian, got Ali to take every known vitamin, but I wouldn't call him a pill-popper," says Angelo Dundee. "That kick lasted for three to four years."

Vitamin deficiency in American athletes is extremely rare. But if it does happen, performance drops dramatically. That's the reason I won't argue against taking a single multivitamin pill to complement your diet. It is the massive overdoses of vitamins that concern me and other physicians.

The current vitamin fad is to take massive overdoses of vitamins C, E, and B_{12}.

Vitamin C

When you exercise or compete, you shouldn't need vitamin C supplements. To keep up with your increased calorie requirements and to avoid chronic fatigue caused by potassium deficiency, you ought to be eating large quantities of fruits and vegetables. There is far more vitamin C in these foods than the athletic body requires. Furthermore, massive doses of vitamin C are negated by the threshold phenomenon. When the blood level of that vitamin exceeds a certain threshold excess, vitamin C spills out into the urine.

Yet many Americans, including athletes and fitness buffs, take vitamin C pills in doses that are frequently from twenty to fifty times their minimal daily requirements.

In 1976, Americans paid $80 million (or 37 cents a person) for vitamin C tablets.

Many vitamin C users have been influenced by Dr. Linus Pauling, winner of two Nobel prizes. He advocates massive doses of vitamin C to prevent colds, cancer, and emotional disease. Dr. Pauling's argument is as follows:

Most mammals don't need vitamin C in their diets because their bodies manufacture it for them. Only man, the gorilla, the guinea pig, and the fruit bat can't manufacture their own vitamin C and therefore must obtain it from their diet.

Using the vitamin C content of bamboo and other vegetables, Professor Pauling computed that a gorilla eats

4,600 milligrams of vitamin C per day. Why then, he asks, are the English told they need only 30 milligrams per day and the Americans told they need only 60 milligrams per day — one-hundredth of what the gorilla eats?

Dr. Pauling has his own answer: "The gorilla eats 4,600 milligrams per day because it is not limited by the Gorilla Council of Nutrition."

He feels that the gorilla has found his optimum intake of vitamin C. After correction for weight differences between man and the gorilla this would work out in man to 2,500 milligrams of vitamin C per day.

The benefits attributed to megadoses of vitamin C have been neither observed nor accepted by most physicians. Pauling's conclusions are theoretical and have not yet been proved by scientifically controlled tests.

Daily doses of up to 1,000 milligrams of vitamin C may be considered to be a vitamin; more than 1,000 milligrams, a drug; and more than 2,000 milligrams, a poison. Before you buy more vitamin C pills, consider the following side effects which, although rare, have been reported in the medical literature.

Diarrhea. This is the single, most common side effect and, according to medical authorities, the chief reason most users become vitamin C dropouts.

Kidney stones. Medical studies report an increase in kidney stones among people who take large amounts of vitamin C.

Decreased fertility. Large amounts of vitamin C act as a contraceptive in men, lowering sperm count. Dosage of more than 2,000 milligrams daily reduces fertility in women.

Abortion. One clinical study shows that sixteen out of twenty pregnant women who took 6,000 milligrams a day of vitamin C aborted in the first few days of pregnancy.

Liver damage. This has been found in experiments with rats, but has not been proved in humans.

Bone fractures. Baby guinea pigs given large doses of vitamin C develop bone fractures.

Drug interaction. Vitamin C blocks the effect of anticlotting agents.

Destruction of B_{12}. Patients taking vitamin C in large quantities may become deficient in vitamin B_{12} — a condition characterized by anemia, nervousness, and weakness. (This side effect is extremely rare.)

Iron poisoning. Vitamin C markedly increases iron absorption, and once in the body, iron can be lost only through bleeding. High iron levels can damage the liver, kidneys, and heart. Pre-menopausal women aren't affected, since they lose blood and iron during menstruation.

Sugar testing. When vitamin C ends up in the urine, it may yield a positive sugar test. This may be mistaken for diabetes.

I can also add my personal experience with vitamin C. In 1965 when I was distance training, I was swallowing 500 to 1,000 milligrams a day. I noticed that every time I omitted vitamin C from my diet, my weekly mileage slipped from a hundred miles to fifty miles. It happened so frequently that I was absolutely convinced my endurance depended on vitamin C.

Then I injured my ankle and was sidelined for two months. Since I wasn't running, I stopped downing vitamin C tablets, and did not resume taking them when I started running again.

My race times were better and my training was certainly as good. I had been quoted in the *Washington Post* as saying that my endurance depended on vitamin C, but now I realized that I had been mistaken.

When you take large doses of vitamin C, your body begins to require it. I had built up a drug dependence. Such dependence has been documented in several studies.

In 1942, during the severe starvation of the thousand-day siege of Leningrad, people from southern Russia who were used to eating fruit regularly developed scurvy — a disease caused by a lack of vitamin C. Northern Russians trapped in Leningrad who never had much vitamin C did not suffer from the disease.

Dr. T. Gordonoff, a Russian physician, found that animals pretreated with vitamin C get scurvy long before animals never given the vitamin. In another report, babies of mothers given large doses of vitamin C during pregnancy developed scurvy early in life. It is normally rare for a baby to get scurvy.

Could Dr. Pauling have made the same mistake that I did? Now that he has taken large doses of vitamin C for an extended period of time, is his body now dependent on these large doses and could he be misinterpreting this dependence for the supposed benefits?

My recommendation is to take your vitamin C where it occurs naturally — in your daily diet. In this way you will not run the risk of side effects from overdosage, and will derive the benefit of other nutrients in the food as well.

Foods High in Vitamin C

Grapefruit
Lemons
Oranges
Strawberries
Tomatoes

Vitamin E

A mystique has grown up around vitamin E that has not been supported by any scientific research done on the human body. In fact the role that vitamin E plays in the human body remains uncertain. To date, the only solid scientific fact that has been established is that vitamin E has value if you are a rat who wants to become pregnant.*

The vitamin E myth started in the 1920s when two researchers. Drs. Herbert M. Evans and Katherine S. Bishop, developed a diet that made some rats vitamin E deficient. The rodents became sterile. When the scientists put vitamin E back in the diet, the rats became fertile again.

Evans and Bishop called their vitamin Tocopherol. In Greek, it means "to bring forth children." Almost immediately it was hailed by physicians and patients alike as a new sexual wonder drug. Athletes jumped on the bandwagon, mistakenly believing that anything that improves potency boosts athletic performance.

Even today some weight lifters take such mammoth doses of vitamin E that it can only be administered by injection. The amount of liquid injected is so large that by the time the shot is finished, the muscle, usually in the buttocks, has increased greatly in size.

Many athletes who tried out for the 1968 Olympic team in the rare atmosphere of Colorado took vitamin E shots. They thought the vitamin would help their tissues hold more oxygen. There is no scientific support for this belief.

Despite the fact that there is no evidence that massive doses of vitamin E confer any benefits, Americans spend $100 million a year on vitamin E capsules.

On the basis of current knowledge, I recommend that you don't take any vitamin E supplements. At best it is a waste of money, and at worst it could be dangerous. Vitamin E in large doses may be toxic. Rats given large amounts develop fat in their arteries and livers. You will get ample vitamin E if you eat a normal diet. It is nearly indestructible, dissolving only in fat, not water, and resists boiling, freezing, and packing. It is found in cereal,

*Vitamin E deficiency does occur in some premature infants who develop a type of anemia and in some people who are unable to absorb fat. It may also help to protect some people with lung disease from some of the adverse effects of air pollution.

margarine, wheat germ, soybeans, and cottonseed and corn oils.

Vitamin B$_{12}$

"The only thing that B$_{12}$ shots do is make your butt sore," says John Lally, the trainer for the Washington Bullets. Yet the only remaining infatuation with vitamins that Muhammad Ali clings to is a vitamin B$_{12}$ shot two days before a fight. Supposedly vitamin B$_{12}$ is another superman-building supplement. Americans fork out millions of dollars for this vitamin every year.

Vitamin B$_{12}$ advocates base their enthusiasm on the work of three Harvard Medical School professors — Drs. George R. Minot, William P. Murphy, and William B. Castle. In the 1920s Minot and Murphy showed that B$_{12}$ dramatically perked up patients with a disease called pernicious anemia.

People with this disease do not have a basic chemical in their stomachs which aids in the absorption of vitamin B$_{12}$ from the foods they eat, as Castle demonstrated. As a result, they become B$_{12}$ deficient. They become weak and tired.

After receiving a B$_{12}$ injection, people with pernicious anemia, who were previously so weak that they couldn't get out of bed, suddenly regained all their vitality. When the general population caught wind of this, taking B$_{12}$ became popular. It's still being taken in large quantities today, even though medical scientists are now convinced that B$_{12}$ helps only those who are deficient in the vitamin. It will not revive people whose tiredness is caused by any other factor.

I've only seen B$_{12}$ deficiency a few times. It's rare because B$_{12}$ is a common vitamin, found in all animal tissue, eggs, and milk. There's none in vegetables, fruits, or grains. Only a pure vegetarian who eats no eggs or dairy products has to worry about getting enough B$_{12}$. The average person can store enough B$_{12}$ to last a decade.

It's sad that in a country like ours, with such good, abundant, varied, and relatively cheap food, people spend hundreds of millions of dollars on vitamins that, for the most part, end up in the sewage system.

8.

Minerals

Why You Need Minerals

Minerals are basic elements found in the soil. They are picked up from the soil by plants. When man eats the plants or animals who have eaten the plants, he incorporates the minerals into his own tissues.

Each mineral has specific functions.

Calcium is the material that makes bones and teeth hard; salt regulates how and where water is distributed in the body; potassium controls muscle heat and nerve conduction. Magnesium regulates muscle contractions and the conversion of carbohydrates to energy.

Some minerals are necessary to form chemicals that regulate body processes: iodine in thyroid hormone, iron in hemoglobin, zinc in insulin, cobalt in vitamin B_{12}, and sulfur in thiamine and biotin.

There are four minerals that the body needs in large amounts and at least fourteen that are needed in trace amounts.

Minerals That the Body Requires

IN LARGE AMOUNTS:

Sodium	Magnesium
Potassium	Calcium

IN TRACE AMOUNTS:

Aluminum	Iodine	Selenium
Boron	Iron	Tin
Chromium	Manganese	Vanadium
Cobalt	Molybdenum	Zinc
Copper	Nickel	

Minerals Required by the Body

MINERAL	SOURCE	RECOMMENDED DAILY ALLOWANCES
Calcium	milk and leafy green vegetables	250 mgm.
Phosphate	milk	750 mgm.
Magnesium	nuts, dark bread, beer, and green leafy vegetables	200 mgm.
Potassium	fruits and vegetables	Not established (requirements increase with exercise)
Manganese	beans	5 mgm.
Iron	raisins	15 mgm.
Copper	beans	2 mgm.
Cobalt	spinach	0.1 mgm.
Iodine	fruits and vegetables grown in coastal areas	.15 mgm.
Sulfur	beans	Not established
Zinc	whole wheat bread	15 mgm.
Fluorine	apples	Not established
Selenium	Fruits and vegetables depending on the selenium content of the soil in which they are grown	.02 mgm.
Chromium	Fruits and vegetables depending on the chromium content of the soil in which they are grown	1 mgm.
Molybdenum	Fruits and vegetables depending on the molybdenum content of the soil in which they are grown	.1 mgm.
Sodium	meat and milk products	2 gm.

Salt (Sodium)

Salt is the most abundant mineral in the blood. Every active person needs salt. If you are low on salt, you may become dehydrated, develop muscle cramps, and not be able to train effectively.

Despite these statements, I recommend that you add as little salt as possible to your food when you are cooking or eating. Why? Because all the salt you need, and more, is contained within the foods you eat: meat, fish, chicken, grains, and nuts are loaded with salt. In 1946 Dr. James

Some Foods That Are High in Salt

All milk products except those advertised as low salt
All margarines except those advertised as low salt
All meats
All fish
All chicken
Olives
Many bran, rye, wheat, and corn products
Salty tasting foods such as sardines, pork, and salted fish
Canned foods that have added salt
Ketchup
Popcorn, potato chips, and french fries
Sauerkraut

Gamble of Harvard Medical School showed that healthy adults can get by with as little as 0.2 grams of salt each day. There is far more salt than this in food you eat. The average American has a daily salt intake of 6 to 18 grams, or sixty times the minimal daily requirement.

I also urge you to throw away your salt pills. Salt tablets make it too easy for you to take in too much salt. Your taste buds regulate the amount of salt you consume. When your body is low on salt, you crave it and will salt your food. When your body has too much salt, you won't like the taste of salt and will avoid it. Salt tablets bypass your taste buds.

The effects of taking too much salt are serious:

Excess salt dehydrates. In low levels, salt helps your body to retain water. But excess body salt increases urination and by drawing more fluid out of the body contributes to heat exhaustion and heatstroke.

Taking excess salt increases potassium loss through the kidneys, which might lead to chronic fatigue.

Too much salt in your blood can cause clotting — leading to a heart attack, stroke, kidney failure, blindness, loss of a limb, or death.

Furthermore, taking too much salt can interfere with the body's ability to retain salt. Training in the heat teaches the kidneys and sweat glands to retain salt. With salt restriction, salt loss through sweat and urine can drop to almost zero. Gulping down excess salt in tablet form negates this process.

The Salt-Restricted Diet

In 1967 the overwhelming favorite for the National AAU 30-kilometer championship (18.6 miles) was Lou Castagnola. I had trained with him the entire year. That winter he broke five national distance records and had won twenty-five consecutive races.

On the day of the race, the weather suddenly turned hot. In a stunning upset, Tom Osler, a mathematician from Glassboro State College in New Jersey, won the race. Three weeks later, in colder weather, Castagnola ran the third fastest marathon ever by an American and Osler was more than ten minutes behind him.

Osler attributed his amazing hot-weather performance to severely restricting salt from his diet. From all I had

Those Who Take Salt Tablets and Those Who Don't

Most athletes who compete in individual sports pass up salt tablets, but many who compete in team sports take them.

Most of the professional teams that we interviewed make salt tablets available. Members of the Buffalo Braves, the Philadelphia Phillies, and the St. Louis Cardinals average one or two salt tablets per player per day. The Boston Celtics dispense 6,000 salt tablets a season, but their trainer says many of these end up on the floor. In hot weather the New York Jets give players four salt tablets the day before a game.

"We don't encourage our players to take salt tablets, but we still go through 3,000 salt tablets a season," says Gene Monahan of the New York Yankees, who doesn't believe there's any benefit in taking them.

John Lally of the Washington Bullets has the best approach: "I don't give salt tablets to the players anymore. If they come to me and ask for them, I explain the side effects and show them the literature."

read about the dangers of salt depletion, I was skeptical. But the mathematics professor knew something that the physicians didn't. By observing his body reactions, Osler discovered that he competed better in hot weather when he restricted salt from his diet.

Dave Costill, a Ball State University physiologist, tested Osler and compared the results with tests on runners who were taking salt. Osler's temperature, heart rate, and amount of sweat were similar to those of other runners. His blood contained comparable amounts of salt. The difference: His sweat and urine contained far less salt. Osler's sweat glands had learned to retain salt.

A few years later, Drs. James Schamadan, William Godfrey, and W. D. Snively in Arizona, and M. Toon in Israel, reported better hot-weather performances in people on a salt-restricted diet.

I have not salted my food for the last ten years. My sweat doesn't taste salty anymore and it doesn't burn when it gets into my eyes.

There is some controversy among physicians whether salt restriction improves performance. If you decide to try salt restriction, observe the following words of caution.

Although salt restriction may help a well-trained athlete, it may increase the chance of injury — perhaps even death — for people who are in poor shape physically. A low salt level interferes with every chemical process in the body — the manufacture of cells, the production of energy, and the circulation of blood.

Don't begin a salt-restriction diet in the summer. Start in the winter to allow your body sufficient time to learn to retain the salt it gets.

Salt restriction is relatively new and should be tried cautiously. If you don't feel well, consult a physician and have blood drawn. If the tests are normal, you will be reassured. If they are abnormal, you may need more salt.

Potassium

Exercisers who feel weak and tired for extended periods may be suffering from mineral blues — a deficiency of the most important minerals inside muscle cells, potassium and magnesium. Of the two, potassium deficiency is more common. Older people and these who take diuretics or who

Eating Foods Rich in Potassium

"The harder I train, the more fruit I eat," says wrestler Dan Gable.

Derek Sanderson says, "I can eat twenty plums at one time."

Golfer Gary Player eats raisins all the time, while Calvin Murphy of the Houston Rockets eats at least ten pieces of fruit a day.

"We order fruits on all our plane rides," says Gene Monahan of the New York Yankees. "On road trips, especially during hot weather, I'll go out and buy four or five bunches of bananas."

"I get fruit for all our players," says Don Seeger of the Philadelphia Phillies. "Pitchers and catchers seem to need it the most."

Tommy Woodcock, the trainer for the St. Louis Blues, serves fruit or juices between periods during hockey games. "Our team goes through three to six dozen oranges a game," he says.

Track coach Brooks Johnson tells his athletes to eat as much fruit as possible.

Muhammad Ali, boxing's superstar, gets his potassium by consuming huge amounts of vegetables.

have diarrhea are more likely to become potassium deficient.

The body has no built-in warning system to signal potassium shortage. Thirst signifies a lack of water. When you are low on salt, you crave salty foods. But when you lack potassium, you just feel tired, weak, and irritable.

Early in my racing career, I reached a period when I couldn't run at all. I was so weak I had difficulty getting out of bed. I previously had run a hundred miles a week, but suddenly a quarter-mile run felt like a marathon. My strength was so low, I thought I was seriously ill.

A simple blood test showed that I was potassium deficient. Downing massive amounts of fruit juices — they are rich in potassium — rejuvenated me.

Many athletes and coaches now recognize that extra potassium is required for exercise. Dr. Ken Rose of the University of Nebraska has found that athletes develop lower blood levels of potassium as the season progresses.

Why do athletes require so much potassium?

Even in frigid temperatures, every muscle that is being exercised produces heat. To keep from overheating, the muscle releases potassium into the bloodstream. This widens the blood vessels, increases blood flow, and carries heat away from the muscle. The potassium is excreted from the body via sweat and urine. Thus an athlete must constantly be on guard to replenish his potassium supply.

Some Foods That Are Rich in Potassium

All fruits	Rye flour
All vegetables	Soybeans
Molasses	Walnuts
Pecans	Wheat germ

Magnesium

Magnesium helps to control muscle contraction and regulates the conversion of carbohydrate to energy. Low levels of magnesium in the muscle cells can cause chronic fatigue and muscle cramps. Magnesium is lost through the stool and sweat. Dr. Kenneth Cooper of the Aerobics Institute in Dallas, Texas, has shown that magnesium is the only mineral whose concentration in the bloodstream is lowered during heavy exercise. A low blood level of magnesium is usually associated with a low muscle level of that mineral.

Dr. Roy J. Shephard of the University of Toronto has demonstrated that distance runners lose substantial amounts of magnesium in their sweat when they run.

A French physician, Dr. B. Boursier, showed that magnesium deficiency was the cause of chronic fatigue in a French soccer team late in their season. He perked them up with magnesium pills.

Some Dietary Sources of Magnesium

Almonds	Oatmeal
Barley	Peanuts
Beans	Peas
Beer	Pecans
Brazil nuts	Rice
Cashew nuts	Soybeans
Cocoa	Green leafy
Corn	vegetables
Dairy products	Walnuts
Hazelnuts	Wheat flour
Meat	

The United States Department of Agriculture reports that 36 percent of the magnesium requirement for Americans is supplied through dairy products and meat. This may be misleading. The calcium in dairy products and the protein in meat may increase your needs for magnesium. Vitamin D supplements and hard alcohol also increase your need for magnesium. Beer is an exception because it contains magnesium and has a relatively low alcohol content.

To avoid magnesium deficiency, eat plenty of dark bread, nuts, and green leafy vegetables, and drink beer in place of other alcoholic beverages.

Calcium

Calcium serves as the main structural material in bones and teeth and is the most abundant mineral in the body. It helps to control muscle contractions and regulates many of the body's chemical reactions.

Except when you are growing, pregnant, or nursing, your calcium requirements are minimal.

When you exercise, your calcium requirements don't increase. You lose almost no calcium in your sweat or urine. The only place you lose calcium is through your stool. If your body needs calcium, it can obtain it from your bones.

A Mineral-Rich Diet

Science has yet to come up with a single pill that contains all the necessary minerals in their proper proportions. It hasn't even done very well with supplying some of the major minerals. Potassium in pill form can cause intestinal ulcers; in liquid form it has a foul taste. Unless bound to protein, magnesium cannot be given in pill form because it is poorly absorbed and can cause diarrhea.

Dolomite pills, which contain potassium and magnesium, are used by some athletes. Several companies have developed commercial drinks for athletes, but most of them contain less potassium and magnesium than orange juice, and no trace elements.

At present the only way you can be sure of getting all the minerals you need, including trace elements, is to eat a

Major Sources of Calcium

Almonds	Figs
Asparagus	Lentils
Beans	Milk
Cabbage	Nuts
Cauliflower	Sardines
Cheese	Turnip greens
Egg yolk	

well-balanced diet. It should contain a wide variety of fruits and vegetables, nuts and grains, and dairy and poultry products.

We cannot expect any particular fruit or vegetable to supply exactly the same mineral content as any other fruit or vegetable, even though it may be of the same type and size. Plants grown in soil deficient in a certain mineral will produce fruits and vegetables that do not contain that mineral. For example, the area around the Great Lakes is known as the goiter belt because its soil is deficient in iodine. A person who eats fruits and vegetables grown only in that area can become deficient in that element and develop an enlarged thyroid gland or goiter if his diet is not supplemented with iodine.

The ideal mineral diet for an athlete would include:

For potassium: A varied diet of fruits and vegetables
For magnesium and trace elements: Various nuts and whole grains
For sodium: Restricted amounts of salt in cooking and eating
For calcium: Low-fat or skim milk and other dairy products

This diet would satisfy the basic mineral needs and is varied enough to provide many of the trace elements as well.

Almost thirty years ago everyone scoffed at Percy Cerutty, the coach of Olympic mile champion and world record holder Herb Elliot. He advocated a diet rich in potassium and magnesium: fruit, vegetables, nuts, and grains. Only in the last few years have scientists caught up with Cerutty.

9.

DRUGS:
Is the Prize Worth the Price?

Do Athletes Take Drugs?

The most effective drug program in sports was developed by Bob Bauman, trainer for the St. Louis Cardinals.

"In 1964, I devised a yellow R.B.I. pill, a red shut-out pill, and a potent green hitting pill," he says. "Virtually every player on the team took them and some wouldn't go out on the field until they took my pills. They worked so well that we won the pennant. We used them again in 1967 and 1968 and also won the pennant.

"They worked because I never told them that the pills were placebos."

The psychological dependence on drugs is the main reason they are used today. Stimulants do not improve athletic performance, but some athletes demand them.

A few years ago I polled more than a hundred top runners and posed this question: "If I could give you a pill that would make you an Olympic champion — and also kill you in a year — would take it?"

To my amazement, more than half of the athletes responding stated that they would take my magic pill. It is this attitude that explains why drug-taking is such a monumental problem in sports today.

Drugs can kill. The first drug death in sports was reported in 1890. A British cyclist died while racing under the influence of ephedrine, a stimulant. There's been little evidence since then to show that stimulants improve athletic performance. Yet athletes continue to take them, and there are needless deaths year after year.

Amphetamine, a stimulant often referred to as an "upper," is by far the most common drug used in sports today. It's part of a national problem, with some 2.2 million Americans using the drug on the theory that it retards fatigue and helps them lose weight.

Actually, amphetamines do not retard or reduce fatigue. They only reduce the *feeling* of fatigue, and mask pain. They can also be habit-forming and can be lethal in combination with hot weather and strenuous competition. Heatstroke, sometimes fatal, is often associated with the use of amphetamines.

The second set of drugs most commonly used in sports are anabolic steroids, hormones that are poorly understood. Many medical authorities and athletes feel that steroids help the body heal itself and some believe they make the body stronger.

According to a U.S. Olympic coach, nearly all the Olympic weight athletes — weight lifters, shot putters, discus throwers — use anabolic steroids.

If athletes take steroids, they must be prepared to pay the price. Known side effects include acne, decreased or increased sexual desire, sterility, dizziness, fainting, headache, lethargy, aggressive behavior, liver disease, bleeding from the intestinal tract, and cancer.

Many top athletes have used drugs at some time in their careers.

"Professional bike racers in Europe complain about drug control in races," Oliver Martin told us. "They feel that the schedule is so hard, they do so much traveling, and are forced to race so often that if they don't take something, they won't be able to compete successfully."

Dave Meggyesy, a former National Football League player, claims in his book, *Out of Their League,* that the league's trainers give drugs to players to boost performance.

Dr. Donald Mandell, a psychiatric consultant to the San Diego Chargers, was threatened with suspension of his medical license because he adminstered amphetamines to the players. He claims he is a scapegoat because he was only trying to wean them off their habit.

Yet every professional team we interviewed, irrespective of the sport, denied the existence of a drug problem. "The rules are so harsh that no trainer gives drugs," says Derek Sanderson. "Jeeze, if I get penicillin for a sore throat, I've got to sign for it in triplicate. Then the trainer gives me only six pills and I've got to sign again just to finish the prescription."

Drugs Banned at the XXI Olympiad at Montreal, Canada, 1976

PSYCHOMOTOR STIMULANT DRUGS

amphetamine
benzphetamine
cocaine
diethylpropion
dimethylamphetamine
ethylamphetamine
fencamfamin
methylamphetamine
methylphenidate
norpseudoephedrine
phendimetrazine
phenmetrazine
prolintane and related compounds

SYMPATHOMIMETIC AMINES

ephedrine
methylephedrine
methoxyphenamine and related compounds

MISCELLANEOUS CENTRAL NERVOUS SYSTEM STIMULANTS

amiphenazole
bemigride
leptazol
nikethamide
strychnine and related compounds

NARCOTIC ANALGESICS

heroin
morphine
methadone
dextromoramide
dipipanone
pethidine and related compounds

ANABOLIC STEROIDS

methandienone
stanozolol
oxymetholone
nandrolone decanoate
nandrolone phenylpropionate and related compounds

SOURCE: Courtesy of the Medical Commission of the International Olympic Committee, Chateau Vidy, Lausanne, Switzerland.

"Most of the players are poor Canadian kids in the National Hockey League who don't even hear of drugs until they come to the United States," says Skip Thayer, trainer for the Chicago Black Hawks. "By that time adults usually do not establish new habits."

"We have a drug education program in professional baseball," says Gene Monahan of the New York Yankees, "and the umpires are alerted to watch for behavioral changes caused by drug-taking."

Dr. Mandell recommends that the National Football League take urine samples of football players on game days on a spot basis. Pete Rozelle, National Football League Commissioner, rejects this suggestion and the National Football League Players Association argues that such a plan amounts to an invasion of privacy.

As far as I could ascertain, no professional teams in any sports are performing urine tests for drugs on a regular basis.

Testing for drugs is complex and expensive. In June 1978, I was the attending physician for the Junior World Bicycle Racing Championships, held in Washington, D.C. Just for this one race, the cost of testing for all drugs would have been about $30,000. It was too expensive to do complete testing.

Amphetamines

European six-day bicycle racers are so competitive that many of them take uppers to compete each day and downers to sleep at night. One English professional bicycle racer had a special kit of two uppers which he self-injected, a downer to get him to sleep at night, and another drug to prevent the other drugs from showing up in his urine.

After Ad Tak, the leading Dutch rider, was disqualified because drugs were detected in his urine, the English cyclist commented, "Ad was caught because his doctor goofed up."

"After a hard day's ride, I saw one cyclist held down by six other professional riders and jabbed in the butt with a syringe full of uppers," reports a professional rider. "He was so high from the injection that he had to ride all night to try to come down. The next morning when all the other riders were 'going up' again, he was 'coming down.'"

The side effects of uppers are well known. Athletes who take amphetamines lose their ability to solve problems. Yet they think they are performing well even when doing poorly.

How the Body Reacts to Amphetamines

JUDGMENT CHANGES

Amphetamine-takers almost always "think" they are performing better than they actually are. They lose the ability to make split-second decisions.

INCREASED SUSCEPTIBILITY TO INJURY

Because amphetamines make one less sensitive to pain, the drug-user doesn't heed pain — nature's warning system. The result: muscle pulls, cramps, and strains. Many heatstroke deaths are directly attributable to amphetamine use.

LONGER RECOVERY TIMES

Football players on amphetamines are still suffering on Tuesday after a Saturday game. Distance runners using the drug have aching muscles up to a week after a race. The normal recovery time: three days.

SYMPTOMS

Users become shaky — like an alcoholic — and suffer from frequent headaches and stomach upsets. Their hearts beat faster and sometimes irregularly — the latter can kill.

MOOD CHANGES

Users become aggressive, hostile, and hyperactive. This is why they are called "uppers." When the drug wears off, depression sets in.

(continued)

Jim Bouton, in his book *Ball Four,* describes the case of a pitcher, under the influence of amphetamine, who refused to be taken out of a ball game because he was "doing so well." He had just delivered three straight home run pitches.

"Amphetamines can do much more harm than good," warns Bob Lundy, trainer for the Miami Dolphins. "I've seen football players in a daze when reporting for practice as late as Tuesday after Sunday's game. Others take them and lose their reactions without realizing it. They may know their assignments perfectly before the game, but when they get in there, they don't know what they're doing. So we don't use them."

"Amphetamines help you to get over your fear of the barbells," asserts Mark Cameron. "But you are not going to lift any more weight than you are capable of lifting so I would never take them."

"Near the end of a long race amphetamines mask fatigue and make a rider feel better than he is supposed to," warns Oliver Martin. "But since amphetamines put such a load on the system, the best athletes will take them only when they are in peak condition."

The army has its own way of teaching about the perils of amphetamines. An old army film shows a recruit traversing an obstacle course in five minutes. After taking amphetamine, he covers the same course in nine minutes, staggers across the finish line elated, and boasts: "I must have broken the course record."

Amphetamine can cause athletes to suffer more than just poor judgment. By masking pain, they increase the chance of injury. Athletes on uppers also require longer periods to recover from endurance events. Amphetamine is habit-forming and can cause severe depression after the initial mood elevation wears off.

They can also be deadly.

Dick Howard, a 1960 Olympic medalist in the hurdles, started on amphetamine to improve his performance. He became hooked on the drug and in 1961 died of an overdose.

Every year I treat dozens of cases of heatstroke, most of them occurring in athletes taking amphetamine. A high school youth died in 1965, because he took an amphetamine before a ten-mile race. That same year, I was unconscious for several hours after racing in 90° heat with amphetamine in my system. At that point I didn't know any better. One wonders how many football deaths in August are due to amphetamine.

HABIT-FORMING

Amphetamines are habit-forming, but not addictive. When a user quits, he can't function properly, can't work, and can't relate well to other people. Thus, the user has a psychological need to return to the drug. The more one uses, the less effective the drug becomes. Therefore, there is a strong tendency to take more of the drug all the time. The ever-increasing doses can lead to more serious side effects and even death.

SOURCE: Gabe Mirkin, M.D.

Tom Simpson, an English cyclist, died under the influence of amphetamine in the 1967 Tour de France. Because many cyclists take amphetamine daily for races that last up to twenty-one days, they have the highest frequency of amphetamine-related deaths.

Psychological Effects of Amphetamines

At hearings before the House Ways and Means Subcommittee on the Trafficking and Control of Narcotics, Barbiturates, and Amphetamines in 1955, it was reported that people on amphetamine are more aggressive and more likely to take criminal action. One can't help wondering if some of the stick-swinging affairs in hockey games are the result of amphetamine use. In the 1974 winter Olympics, the Czechoslovakian hockey team was disqualified because drugs were found in the urine of one of its players.

In 1966, G. A. Talland and G. C. Quarton demonstrated that amphetamine can improve performance, but only when taken regularly by people performing a simple, uncomplicated task.

But it has been proved repeatedly that amphetamine impairs performance in a sport like football that requires split-second problem solving. Because of this, many football coaches will not allow their athletes to take amphetamine pills. Nor will any coach of an athlete who competes in any event requiring skill.

"I've never heard of a gymnast taking amphetamine," says former Olympic gymnast Greg Weiss.

"All amphetamine would do is mess up your coordination," says Butch Buchholz, the commissioner of World Team Tennis.

In June 1957, a resolution was presented to the American Medical Association to condemn the use of stimulants in athletic events. Dr. Peter Karpovich, a professor at Springfield College, and Drs. Henry K. Beecher and W. Smith of Harvard Medical School were commissioned to study the effects of stimulants on athletic performance.

Dr. Karpovich found amphetamine to be of no benefit. However, Beecher and Smith reported that amphetamine slightly improved the performance of runners, weight lifters, discus throwers, and swimmers.

Dr. William Pierson, a physiologist in Los Angeles, used the Beecher-Smith data and came to the opposite conclusion. His interpretation was published in the *Journal of the American Medical Association.*

Where did Beecher and Smith go wrong? Some of the runners timed themselves, and the throwers did not take exact measurements. Because amphetamine makes the athlete feel he is performing better than he actually is, the slight improvement reported in the Beecher-Smith study could be attributed to the athletes' own impressions.

Indeed, after Dr. Pierson's letter appeared in the *Journal,* Drs. Beecher and Smith published a second paper dealing with the psychological effects of amphetamines on athletes. They also concluded this time that athletes under the influence of the drug felt they ran faster and threw farther than the stopwatch and tape measure recorded. One runner was absolutely elated by his performance even though it was well below his usual standards. Thus a close scrutiny of both studies shows that amphetamines do not boost athletic performance.

Several other studies since then have failed to show that amphetamines improve any athlete's performance.

If the effects of uppers are so obviously bad, why do athletes continue to use them?

The answer lies in the constant search for a short cut to high performance — a miracle drug to turn us all into supermen.

I was a single-time user of amphetamines, and it almost cost me my life. I want to emphasize to all athletes — particularly those with tremendous drive to excel — that taking amphetamines is not the route to success, and can be the path to destruction.

Anabolic Steroids

Since the stress of prolonged exercise results in tissue damage, quicker healing means quicker recovery time and ultimately more time for training and muscle building. Anabolic steroids have a reputation for aiding this process.

Guy Borrelli, a national-champion weight lifter, recalls injuring his hamstring muscle in a professional football game ten years ago. "The trainer," he said, "injected me with anabolic steroids and the muscle healed in a week instead of the usual month."

Most sportsmedicine physicians can't agree among themselves whether anabolic steroids help to make the athlete stronger. Yet virtually all champion weight lifters are convinced that anabolic steroids are strength builders.

Almost all champion weight lifters take anabolic steroids at some time in their competitive lives, according to several coaches. So pervasive has the practice become that professional, college, and even high school football coaches routinely dispense steroids. Their use is also very common in other sports requiring muscle strength: the weight events in track and field, wrestling, and karate.

Anabolic steroids are produced in small amounts by the healthy body, and apparently function in some way to heal damaged tissue. Artificial steroids were originally given to people who were unable to produce their own because they had such disorders as severe burns, disseminated cancer, malnutrition, and severe weight loss.

Most scientists feel that additional doses of anabolic steroids don't help to increase tissue in a person who produces normal amounts of the hormones.

Dr. G. H. Hervey of the University of Leeds (England) writes: "The more positive consensus is that if anabolic steroids are taken during training, fatigue is retarded and the amount of work done per session increases. The additional training is thought to provide the real benefit."

Most scientific studies show that laboratory rats (and, for that matter, novice weight lifters) do not become stronger when they take anabolic steroids. For example, members of a college physical education class or a YMCA class do not benefit from steroids because they are not working at maximum capacity. They never tire their bodies enough to need the shorter recovery periods anabolic steroids help provide.

It is the increased work done, then, and not just the pill, that makes athletes stronger.

The benefits of steroid-taking only accrue to highly motivated and knowledgeable strength athletes involved in top-flight competition.

Dick Drescher, the former University of Maryland track star and Pan American games discus champion, raises important questions about Communist Bloc sovereignty in weight events in track and field.

He notes that Americans used to be the best in weight events until the advent of anabolic steroids. Then the Russian and European athletes were taught by their physicians how to use anabolic steroids effectively. According to Drescher, American athletes are just groping in the dark. He claims athletes don't know which pills to

Position Statement of the American College of Sports Medicine on the Use of Anabolic Steroids by Athletes

Based on a comprehensive survey of the world literature and a careful analysis of the claims made for and against the efficacy of anabolic-androgenic steroids in improving human physical performance, it is the position of the American College of Sports Medicine that:

1. The administration of anabolic-androgenic steroids to healthy humans below age 50 in medically approved therapeutic doses often does not of itself bring about any significant improvements in strength, aerobic endurance, lean body mass, or body weight.

2. There is no conclusive scientific evidence that extremely large doses of anabolic-androgenic steroids either aid or hinder athletic performance.

3. The prolonged use of oral anabolic-androgenic steroids (C_{17}-alkylated derivates of testosterone) has resulted in liver disorders in some persons. Some of these disorders are apparently reversible with the cessation of drug usage, but others are not.

4. The administration of anabolic-androgenic steroids to male humans may result in a decrease in testicular size and function and a decrease in sperm production. Although these effects appear to be reversible when small doses of steroids are used for short periods of time, the reversibility of the effects of large doses over extended periods of time is unclear.

(continued)

take, how many to take, how long to stay with them, or how long to stay off them.

Ironically, at the 1976 Olympics, two American weight lifters were disqualified because traces of anabolic steroids were found in their urine. The urine tests were described by a top American lifter this way:

"It was a joke. First of all the test was hit or miss. Most lifters weren't tested. Some lifters who passed the urine test admitted to me that they had been using steroids until a few days before the Olympic competition."

Indeed, out of the thousands of athletes in the Montreal Olympics, only 166 athletes in eight different sports were tested for steroids. According to several Olympic athletes, it was common knowledge in the Olympic village that the Russian lifters had been given medication that masked steroid usage.

For many years medical scientists have been able to mask the excretion of drugs in the urine. Horse trainers, for example, have given horses a drug called Lasix to prevent other prohibited drugs from being detected in the urine. Physicians do the same thing. For example, in treating gonorrhea, they use probenecid, a drug that prevents penicillin from entering the urine, keeping a high level of it in the bloodstream.

Alexeev, the Russian Olympic super-heavy weight lifting champion, was ordered to report for a urine test five days before competition. He didn't supply a urine sample until the day of the competition. Could he have needed the extra days to clear his urine of a drug?

Members of the United States team were openly hostile about the disqualification of the two American lifters at the 1976 Olympics. They felt that everyone should have been tested.

"By slapping a few athletes on the wrist, the true controversy over anabolic steroids was covered up," one lifter said.

In 1975, the International Federation of Sports and Medicine brought together leading physicians from many countries for a symposium on anabolic steroids. Even though studies done on highly competitive weight lifters usually show that anabolic steroids were effective, the members of the symposium concluded: "Anabolic steroids in healthy, young athletes are not fully understood. Studies show conflicting results of increase in strength and improvement in performance."

Several explanations can be offered for the reluctance of the symposium members to endorse anabolic steroids.

5. Serious and continuing efforts should be made to educate male and female athletes, coaches, physical educators, physicians, trainers, and the general public regarding the inconsistent effects of anabolic-androgenic steroids on improvement of human physical performance and the potential dangers of taking certain forms of these substances, especially in large doses, for prolonged periods.

SOURCE: From *Medicine and Science in Sports*, volume 8, no. 2, pp. xi–xii, 1976. Copyright 1976, the American College of Sports Medicine. Reprinted by permission.

Studies yield conflicting results.

There is no effective means to do a double-blind study in which the weight lifters do not know whether they are on a placebo or steroids. All champion weight lifters can tell when they are on steroids.

Yet it is impossible to police international competition. No test has been devised which can detect steroids more than a few weeks after the last pill has been taken.

As is shown in the chart, anabolic steroids can cause several side effects.

Many coaches do not understand the consequences of giving young players steroids. Many youngsters do not stop growing until they are out of their teens. Medical scientists have known for many years that anabolic steroids cause premature closure of the epiphyses of growing bones and stop growth forever.

While most athletes on anabolic steroids experience no noticeable side effects, some scientists feel that long-term use of anabolic steroids may predispose an athlete to a future heart attack, cancer, or sterility.

Although most athletes do not want to take steroids, many feel compelled to do so in order to be able to compete effectively.

Mr. A. H. Payne, an authority on weight lifing at England's University of Birmingham, says, "The majority of athletes I have spoken to . . . would welcome drug tests if they would insure that no drug taken in the world can escape detection. The athletes themselves, on the whole, want to come off steroids."

Indeed it is unfortunate that most athletes competing at the international level in events requiring strength are forced to buy present accomplishments with the possible sacrifice of future health.

The Side Effects of Anabolic Steroids

BODY EFFECTS

Damages the liver (hepatitis)
May cause liver cancer
Causes atrophy of the testicles
Causes bleeding from the intestinal tract
May increase one's chances for a future heart attack
May cause temporary sterility. Almost 100 percent of males who take anabolic steroids for more than eight weeks have decreased sperm counts.
Masculinizes the female by stimulating growth of hair on the face, legs, and abdomen
Causes or aggravates acne
Makes the voice hoarse and raspy
Stops growth in young athletes

SYMPTOMS

Increased or decreased sexual desire
Fainting and dizziness
Headache
Lethargy
Aggression

LABORATORY FINDINGS

Increases fat levels in the bloodstream, magnifying the chance of a heart attack
Increases blood pressure
Occasionally causes abnormal liver function
Causes abnormal rise in blood sugar

SOURCE: Gabe Mirkin, M.D.

10.

Common Injuries and What to Do about Them

This chapter is about the aches, pains, strains, and sprains that you will encounter from time to time in your athletic career. Many such injuries heal by themselves without medical supervision, but some of them, if left untreated, can hamper or even end your participation in a sport.

It is not the intention of this chapter to make you into a sportsmedicine physician, but rather to give you insight and understanding about several common and important injuries.

When to See a Doctor

You should consult a physician for:

1. All traumatic joint injuries. All injuries to a joint and its ligaments should be examined by a sportsmedicine physician because these injuries have the potential of becoming permanent and debilitating if proper treatment is not administered. In the meantime, to prevent further damage, keep the injured joint as immobile as possible.

2. Any injury accompanied by severe pain. Pain is nature's way of talking to you and when it speaks loudly, you had better listen.

3. Any pain in a joint or bone that persists for more than two weeks. These tissues are the ones in which the most serious injuries occur.

4. Any injury that doesn't heal in three weeks. All injuries that don't heal should be checked for a structural

Household Words

Athletic injuries are so common that their names are everyday household words: tennis elbow, runner's knee, sprinter's shins, jumper's knee, halfback's hamstring, wrestler's ear, and swimmer's shoulder.

abnormality that may have caused them. Sometimes an injury may not heal because you won't rest it.

5. Any injury that you feel should be checked. If you are concerned about an injury, you should always ask for help. Your own intuition may be superior to anything that I write in a book.

6. Any infection in or under the skin manifested by pus, red streaks, swollen lymph nodes, or fever. Untreated infections may lead to serious complications, and since antibiotics generally bring relief quickly, it is foolish not to receive treatment.

I would emphasize that these six rules are, at best, rough guidelines designed to save you from unnecessary medical bills and perhaps unnecessary treatment. It must be realized, however, that every injury is a happening unto itself and should be treated on its own merits, not strictly by guidelines in a book.

What to Do First

The immediate treatment for almost all athletic injuries is the same, whether you've pulled a muscle, strained a ligament, hurt a joint, or broken a bone. It's a four-part program that you can follow even if you will be seeking a physician's advice and it is abbreviated RICE:

Rest: Rest is necessary because continued exercise or other activity could extend the injury. Stop using the injured part the minute it is hurt.

Ice: Ice decreases the bleeding from injured blood vessels because it causes them to contract. The more blood that collects in a wound, the longer it takes to heal.

Compression: Compression limits swelling which, if uncontrolled, could retard healing. Following trauma, blood and fluid from the surrounding tissues leak into the damaged area and distend the tissue. Swelling is sometimes useful since it brings antibodies to kill germs, but if the skin is not broken, antibodies are unnecessary and swelling only prolongs healing.

Elevation: Elevation of the injured part to above the level of the heart uses the force of gravity to help drain excess fluid.

Because swelling usually starts within seconds of an injury, start RICE as soon as possible. First place a towel over the injured area. Then apply an ice pack, ice chips, or cubes over the towel. Do not apply the ice directly to the skin as it can cause the skin to hurt.

For compression, wrap an elastic bandage firmly over the ice, around the injured part. Be careful not to wrap the area so tightly that you shut off the blood supply. The signs of a shut-off blood supply are numbness, cramping, and pain. If any of these happens, unwrap the area immediately. Otherwise, leave the ice pack and bandage in place for thirty minutes. Next, to allow the skin to rewarm and the blood to recirculate, unwrap the area for fifteen minutes. Then rewrap the area. Repeat this procedure for three hours. If the area continues to swell or the pain increases, check immediately with a physician if you have not already done so.

If the injury is severe, you can follow the RICE program for up to twenty-four hours. If pain and swelling persist forty-eight hours after the injury, apply heat. Further treatment depends on the type of tissue that was injured.

How to Tell What Has Been Injured

I treat athletes according to their injuries, not the sport they play. A hamstring pull is treated in the same manner whether it occurs in a football player or a runner. For each of the six internal tissue structures of the body most frequently involved in sports injuries, the same principles apply. These six tissue structures are:

Muscles	Joints, including cartilage
Tendons	Ligaments
Bones	Fasciae

A seventh tissue, the skin, commonly subject to injury is external. Except for skin injuries, which are visible, it is often hard to tell which tissue in particular has been injured unless you understand and apply basic anatomy. For example, if it hurts to touch or move your ankle, knee, hip, wrist, elbow, or shoulder, you probably have a joint, ligament, or cartilage injury. If your muscle, the soft fleshy mass under your skin, hurts when you move or touch it, you have a muscle injury. The same goes for the tendon, the long, narrow and tough fiber that extends out from the muscle. Injuries to the fasciae, fibrous sheets that surround and protect muscles, tendons, and organs, are difficult to diagnose by a nonphysician. Bone injuries are probably the most painful of all injuries. Moving or touching a broken bone will be extremely painful.

How Long Will It Take You to Recover?

The time it takes your injury to heal depends on several factors:

Whether you received adequate early treatment (RICE).
Your level of conditioning when you were injured. The better shape you're in, the quicker you heal.
How badly you're injured. The more extensive the injury, the longer it takes to heal.
Whether you rested the injured tissue long enough for it to heal.

When Can You Resume Your Sport?

To be a successful athlete, you must learn to read your body's signals. If the injured part hurts at rest, you should not exercise it.

As soon as your injured part stops hurting at rest, you can exercise it minimally. That means *slowly.* And as soon as you can exercise without pain, you can start to increase the workload and intensity. If the pain returns, cut back the intensity of your workout. I will cover this in more detail when we talk about each specific injury.

In the meantime, you should do some activity to maintain your cardiovascular fitness. Perform some other exercise that will not involve the injured part.

For example, if the bottom of your foot hurts so that you can't run, ride a bike. If your shoulder aches, try to jog. If you have pain in your leg, pull on a rowing machine. Remember, it doesn't take long to lose cardiovascular fitness. You will gain much more from exercising than from sitting in a hot bath or resting in bed.

Muscles

The term *muscle* comes from the Latin word for mouse. Like a mouse, a muscle has a body, which is the muscle itself, and a tail, which is the tendon. The tendon acts as an extension of the muscle and in most cases attaches onto a bone.

Muscles are the motors that move every part of the body. You can't talk, breathe, eat, or blink without using your muscles. All muscles produce movement by the same method. By shortening, they pull on their tendons or attachments which, in turn, move bones. For example, when the biceps, which is on the front of your upper arm, contracts, the forearm is brought toward your body.

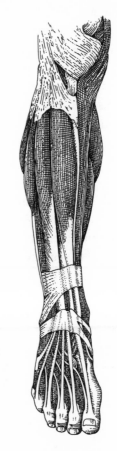

Muscles and Their Tendons
(*Dark area is muscle, white is tendon.*)

Muscle Soreness

At one time or another, everyone experiences muscle soreness, which usually sets in eight to twenty-four hours after exercise. If the discomfort is very localized, the muscle may be injured to some degree. However, all muscle soreness is not due to injury. If the soreness is diffuse, it is probably the result of swelling of the muscle fibers, which are stretched with each muscle contraction. Such soreness is very common. On days when you are sore, exercise at a relaxed pace. On the following day, you will usually feel better and will be able to exercise intensely again.

There is no medical treatment for soreness. Many athletes apply a liniment containing oil of wintergreen, a concentrated solution similar to aspirin. This liniment alleviates pain, but it does not hasten healing.

Even if you are in top physical shape, you can develop soreness in the muscles you don't use often. For example, I've run for thirty years. But last spring after painting my barn, my arms were so sore I couldn't lift them. I was using my arm muscles differently from when I run.

Pulled Muscles

A pulled muscle is an acute tear of muscle fibers and is characterized by sudden, localized and persistent pain in a muscle that is being stressed. The sprinter gets it in the hamstring, the swimmer in the shoulder, and the jockey in the inner thigh muscles. Even though there are more than five hundred muscles, less than 5 percent are commonly injured.

When a muscle starts to tear, it will really hurt. When you develop a sudden sharp pain in a muscle, stop exercising immediately. If you attempt to continue exercising, you will cause further damage to the muscle fibers and prolong the healing time.

Causes

Muscle pulls result when more tension is applied to a muscle than it can bear. As a general rule, the more severe the pain, the more extensive the injury. Usually muscle pulls occur when you try to exercise intensely at a time when one or more of the following factors predispose you to injury:

Insufficient warm-up. Your muscles are stiff and tight and therefore susceptible to injury. Before playing a sport you should warm up for at least ten minutes by performing that sport with slow, easy movements and gradually increase the pace. (See "Warming Up," in Chapter 11.)

Poor flexibility. Every time you exercise hard, your muscles are slightly damaged. With healing, they shorten and, like a tight violin string, are more susceptible to tearing unless you have restored flexibility by stretching. (See "Lack of Flexibility," in Chapter 11.)

Overtraining. Every time you exercise intensely, your muscles suffer slight damage. If you exercise intensely again before your muscles have had time to heal, you are much more likely to injure them. (See "The Overtraining Syndrome," in Chapter 11.)

Muscle imbalance. Every muscle that moves a limb in one direction has an opposing muscle that moves it in the other direction. If one muscle is much stronger than the other, it can overpower and damage the weaker one. (See "Muscle Imbalance," in Chapter 11.)

Mineral deficiency. Lack of sodium, potassium, magnesium, and other minerals can predispose to muscle injury. (See Chapter 8.)

Structural abnormality. Certain structural abnormalities, such as flat feet, unequal arm or leg length, or a deep curve in the back, have the effect of putting excess stress on a particular muscle and make that muscle more likely to be injured. For instance, if one leg is shorter than the

Muscle Pull

Going into the last event of the 1977 United States–Russia Track and Field Meet, the United States men's team appeared to have won. They already had more points than the Russians and were heavily favored in the mile relay. In the last lap, Maxie Parks, the United States anchorman, had a commanding lead when he suddenly and tragically pulled up lame in severe pain with a torn hamstring. The Russian runner passed him and won the meet for his team.

other, the muscles of the longer leg are more prone to injury. (See "Structural Abnormalities," in Chapter 11.)

Poor training methods. All training programs should include gradual increases in workload, speed, and resistance. Rapid increases in these factors often lead to more stress than a muscle can handle and result in an injury. (See "Poor Training Methods," in Chapter 11.)

Trauma. Stepping into a hole or being hit by someone can cause excess muscle stress and consequent injury.

Lack of an adequate endurance program. Rhythmic endurance exercises thicken the muscles, tendons, and ligaments and make them more resistant to injury. Every athlete should have a year-round exercise program for the muscles he or she uses in competition.

Treatment

There is no medication that will make your muscle heal faster. The immediate treatment for a muscle pull is RICE.

Discontinue the ice and compression in twenty-four hours or less. If the ice causes the skin to hurt, stop the ice treatment at that time. As long as there is swelling, elevation should be continued.

Most physicians and trainers recommend the use of heat forty-eight hours after the pull has occurred. Heat dilates the blood vessels and increases the blood supply, which brings increased amounts of nutrients to the injured area. Nutrients are the muscle's building blocks and also provide energy for healing. Heat may possibly increase the rate of the healing process itself.

The long-term treatment is to strengthen the injured muscle so that it will stand up better to stress.

When to start exercising again

Most pulled muscles heal in two to fourteen days. The older you are, the longer it takes to heal. With age, every process in the body slows down.

Wait until your muscle stops hurting at rest before you try to exercise. Then exercise at a relaxed pace. If you're a runner, don't try to run hard until you can jog without pain. If you're a swimmer with an injured shoulder, don't try to swim fast intervals until you can swim leisurely without pain. If you're a tennis player with an elbow injury, don't try to play tennis until you can swing the racket without pain.

Realize that the pulled muscle will always feel tight when it is healing because the healing process causes it to shorten. For example, after a hamstring pull, you will not be able to touch your toes even though you were able to do so before you were injured. By doing gentle stretching exercises, gradually building up your workload, and slowing down every time your muscles hurt, you will eventually be able to train at the same level as before your injury, and your muscles will be as good as new.

Tennis Elbow

Tennis elbow is usually caused by excessive strain on the muscles of the forearm which attach at the elbow. These muscles produce forward and backward movement at the wrist.

The pain is usually where the muscles attach below the elbow joint.* Tennis players suffer from two types of tennis elbow:

Forehand tennis elbow — common in professional players — which stems from the wrist snap in booming serves. Serving strains the muscles that bend the wrist. These muscles attach on the inner side of the elbow and consequently the pain occurs at this site.

Backhand tennis elbow — common in novice or weekend players — comes from hitting backhand strokes incorrectly. A backhand stresses the muscles that straighten the wrist. These muscles attach on the outer side of the elbow.

"I've yet to see tennis elbow in a player with a two-handed backhand," reports Dr. Arthur Bernhang of the State University of New York. "Evidently using two hands protects the elbow muscles, tendons, and ligaments from too much force."

People who try to hit the ball with a wrist movement rather than using their entire upper arm are generally more susceptible to tennis elbow. A wrist swing puts tremendous stress on the muscles of the forearm. It follows, therefore,

Tennis Elbow (Muscle Injury)

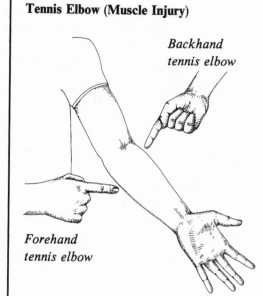

Backhand tennis elbow

Forehand tennis elbow

---

*Athletes can also injure the tendons of the upper arm which attach at the elbow. In this condition, the pain occurs just above the elbow joint. It is due to rotating or turning the arm in or out. Pitchers and bowlers who throw curves often suffer from this condition. Like all other tendon injuries, it is treated by stretching the tendon.

that the stronger your forearm muscles, the more protected you are from this condition.

Here are some additional factors that put added stress on the muscles, tendons, and joints and that may result in tennis elbow:

Using too heavy a racket. The heavier the racket, the more stress on the arm.

Playing on grass or cement. The ball bounces off these surfaces with a greater velocity, hitting the racket with a greater force, which is transmitted to the elbow.

Using heavy balls. The heavier the ball, the greater the force against the racket.

Having too much tension on the strings. If the strings are too tight, they do not give sufficiently when the ball hits and a greater force is transmitted to the elbow.

Using an oversize grip. If the racket is held insecurely, the ball will be hit with a wobbly stroke and the elbow absorbs the shock.

Some physicians feel that an aluminum racket is superior to a wooden one because it bends more when the ball hits it. Wooden rackets are stiffer.

However, some tennis players report that aluminum rackets recoil after the initial impact and hurt their elbows even more. Regardless of the type of tennis racket you use, if you develop tennis elbow, hitting the tennis ball will aggravate the condition.

Interestingly, you don't even have to play tennis to develop tennis elbow. Bowler Don Carter, cross-country skier Tim Caldwell, and pitcher Bob Gibson have all suffered from tennis elbow.

It can come from any motion that turns the wrist or stresses the elbow. The housewife may get it from opening jars; the carpenter from turning his screwdriver; the bowler and pitcher from flicking the wrist when releasing the ball; and the cross-country skier from pushing off on his ski poles.

The treatment of tennis elbow is the same regardless of its cause: rest followed by strengthening the injured muscles. No other treatment is effective.

How can you avoid tennis elbow? Most amateur players have an improper grip and a poor stroke which contribute to this condition. A few tennis lessons can improve a novice player's technique and can strengthen the muscles before they become injured.

Wrist Hitters

Rod Laver, Tony Roche, Arthur Ashe, and I all ended up with tennis elbow. We hit the ball primarily with our wrists. This puts tremendous force on our elbows.

Pancho Gonzales, Ken Rosewall and Pancho Segura were immune to tennis elbow. They hit the ball from the shoulder down.

— BUTCH BUCHHOLZ,

Buchholz himself, a many-time U.S. Davis Cup player and Commissioner of World Team Tennis, had to retire at the height of his career because of tennis elbow. He submitted to twenty anti-inflammatory steroid shots (cortisone) and now has trouble lifting a suitcase.

Exercises for the Prevention and Treatment of Tennis Elbow

When you first develop pain in your elbow, stop playing tennis. After waiting two to seven days for the pain to disappear, start the following exercises. Perform each twice a day.

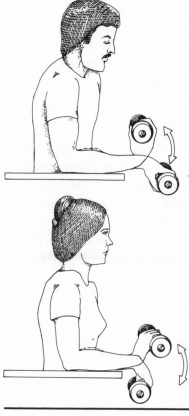

For forehand tennis elbow: Lay your arm flat on a table, letting your hand extend over the edge, your palm facing up. With a five-pound weight, flex your wrist ten times. Repeat until you tire.

For backhand tennis elbow: Lay your arm flat on a table, letting your hand extend over the edge, your palm facing down. With a five-pound weight, flex your wrist ten times. Repeat until you tire.

Muscle Cramps

Muscle cramps are painful, sustained contractions of all of the fibers in a muscle. They can last for just a few seconds or continue for several hours.

Any muscle can cramp. The cramp can be so mild that you will feel only a slight muscle twitch or so severe that it can break a bone. Although cramps can occur during sleep, they usually occur during intense exercise. No athlete or fitness buff in any sport is immune to this common condition.

There are many causes:

Salt deficiency
Low levels of other minerals such as potassium or magnesium
An injury or strain on the muscle

A Muscle Cramp That Almost Cost $25,000

What would you do if you were in the last three laps of a 500-mile automobile race worth thousands of dollars and your leg suddenly began to cramp? Buddy Baker describes his experience in the 1976 Winston 500 in Talladega, Alabama.

"The pain was horrible and my whole leg went into spasm, but I didn't take my foot off the pedal." His tenacity won the race by less than half a car length and he collected more than $25,000 in prize money.

Many soccer players on the Dallas Tornado suffered from frequent muscle cramps until the team superstar, Kyle Rote, Jr., persuaded them to eat large amounts of bananas for potassium and other minerals. The players haven't been plagued by cramps in recent years.

An obstruction of the muscle's blood supply by sustained muscular contractions

Hyperventilating — breathing too fast when it is not necessary, which prevents the body from using calcium

In my opinion, the most common cause of cramps in athletes is a low body level of one or more minerals, particularly potassium and salt. Potassium is the mineral that is lost in large amounts during hard exercise.

I suggest that you eat more fruits and vegetables to replace potassium. I do not recommend that you increase your dietary intake of salt even though several medical texts make this recommendation. Years ago when I was taking salt tablets and salting my food heavily, I frequently would get muscle cramps in hot weather. However, for the last ten years I have severely restricted salt from my diet and have not had any muscle cramps. Many of my marathon-running friends have had the same experience. It is my opinion that when an athlete consumes large amounts of salt, his body loses its ability to conserve salt. Consequently, if he suddenly decreases his salt intake, his salt level will become unusually low and this will cause cramps.

If you still continue to have cramps in spite of an increased intake of mineral-rich foods, see your physician. He will draw blood for an analysis of your mineral levels. If your levels are abnormal, he will recommend certain foods to replenish the minerals in your body. But if the tests are normal, you still could be deficient in potassium or magnesium. Since potassium and magnesium are found primarily inside the cells, blood tests are not always an accurate measure of the body's level of the two minerals. The best way to measure these minerals is to cut out a piece of muscle and measure the amount of minerals inside it. However, because the treatment of mineral deficiency is so simple — eating fruits, vegetables, and grains — a muscle biopsy is never necessary.

Stitches

Causes

Stitches, the sudden, sharp pains that athletes sometimes experience in the upper part of the abdomen, are a form of muscle cramp. Physicians now feel that most stitches are due to a cramp of the diaphragm — the large flat muscle

Treatment of a Calf Cramp

The treatment of a cramp is to stretch and squeeze the muscle. If it's the calf, squeeze the muscle with one hand and stretch it by pushing the front part of the foot up with the other. If it's the biceps, squeeze the muscle with one hand and have a colleague straighten the elbow.

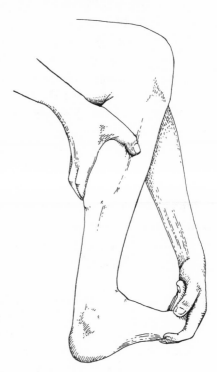

that controls breathing. The cramp is caused by the blood supply to the diaphragm being shut off by pressure from the lungs above and the abdomen below. When you breathe hard, your lungs fill up with air and push down on the diaphragm. When you run, you raise your legs with each step. To do this you must contract your belly muscles. This decreases the size of your abdominal cavity, which, in turn, exerts a pressure from below on the diaphragm. The dual pressure closes down the blood supply and the muscle, being unable to get enough oxygen, goes into a spasm.

Another cause of stitch, particularly in novice athletes, is gas distending the colon. The colon makes up the last three feet of the intestinal tract and functions as a muscular tube which moves stool toward the rectum.

As a result of the degradation of food, gas is formed throughout the entire intestinal tract. Exercise speeds up intestinal contractions and pushes gas toward the rectum. That's why athletes often pass gas during exercise.

If the flow of gas is blocked by hard stools, the colon is stretched like a balloon and a stitch occurs. The most common place for this obstruction is the right upper part of the abdomen, where there is a bend in the colon.

There are other causes of stitches:

Eating just before you exercise. When you exercise, large amounts of blood must be pumped to your muscles. When food is in your stomach, blood must be pumped to your intestinal tract to aid digestion. If there is not enough oxygen to supply your muscles, blood flow to your intestinal tract is diminished and you can develop intestinal cramps.

An intolerance to milk or wheat. There are people who lack the enzyme chemicals in their intestinal tract that break down either a sugar in milk, called galactose, or a protein in wheat, called glutin. When people who lack one of these enzymes eat the corresponding food, they may develop cramping or diarrhea. However, some of these people develop cramping only when they exercise vigorously within twenty-four hours of eating these foods.

Prevention and cure

If you develop stitches frequently, be sure you don't eat for three to five hours before exercising. If that doesn't work, try avoiding milk for forty-eight hours. If that fails, avoid wheat products for the same length of time.

Cramping of your diaphragm is prevented by strengthening your diaphragm and belly muscles. To strengthen your diaphragm, run fast two or more times a week. To strengthen your belly muscles, do bent-knee sit-ups (see diagram on page 115).

The best way to prevent the stitch caused by a distended colon is to soften the stool so that the gas can pass unobstructed. Since a diet rich in starch yields a hard stool and a diet heavy in fruits and vegetables yields the opposite, you should eat less bread, potatoes, and spaghetti, and more fruits and vegetables.

What should you do when you get a stitch? Slow down and push your fingers deep into the site of the pain, usually just below the last rib on the right upper part of your belly. Bend forward and exhale, pursing your lips. The pain will disappear soon and you can continue running. When you get a stitch, it is not necessary to see a doctor.

Starchy Food Forms Claylike Stool

To better understand how foods affect the consistency of your stool, consider the difference between clay and sand. Sand is soft because it is comprised of very large particles that do not stick together. Clay is hard because it is comprised of very small particles that *do* stick together. Starchy foods break down to form very small particles and yield a hard stool. Fruits and vegetables break down to form large fibers and yield a soft stool.

Tendons

Tendons are strong fibrous bands that attach muscles to bone. To understand better what a tendon is, find the wide part of your calf muscle in the middle part of the back of your lower leg. The tendon starts where the wide calf muscle suddenly becomes a narrow band above your heel. This is your Achilles tendon. With your hand, follow the band down to where it attaches to the back of your heel bone.

Muscles and tendons are an integral unit. Tendons, which are ropelike extensions of the muscles, do not contract. Only muscles do. For example, when the calf muscle contracts, it pulls the Achilles tendon up, which in turn pulls the front part of the foot down. When muscles are shortened by hard exercise, the tension of the muscle–tendon complex is increased.

Tendons are more susceptible to injury than muscles for two reasons:

Tendons have a smaller cross section than muscles, which means they don't have as large an area over which force can be distributed. As a result, there is more strain on tendons than on muscles during exercise.

Tendons are located in areas where they can be injured easily. When they move, they may rub against bones, ligaments, and other tendons. On the other hand, muscles are located in protected areas. They never rub against other rough tissue.

Calf Muscle and Achilles Tendon

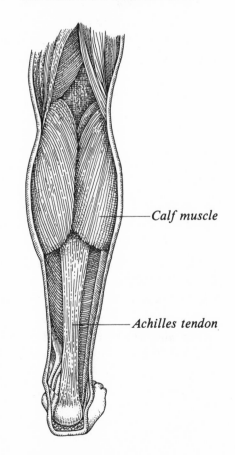

— Calf muscle

— Achilles tendon

Tendon Rupture

A tendon rupture is a separation of a tendon from a bone or muscle, or a complete tear in the tendon itself. Bone and muscle separations are the most common tendon ruptures.

Cause

Tendon ruptures are usually the result of sudden violent contractions. They occur in sprinters, handball players, weight lifters, and athletes in other sports where sudden bursts of speed are required. Athletes who have tight, inflexible muscles are obviously most susceptible to tendon ruptures.

When an athlete ruptures his tendon, you generally can hear the pop. The pain is so severe that the athlete usually writhes in pain and holds the affected muscle in a contracted position. He will not let it be moved and usually won't even let it be examined unless he first receives pain medicine. If the tendon is in the leg, the athlete usually is carried off on a stretcher. If a tendon rupture is suspected, consult a physician immediately. In the meantime, apply RICE.

The area over the tendon becomes swollen and usually hurts for days. After a day or two, a huge black and blue mark from the internal bleeding appears on the skin overlying the rupture. By sending out fibrous filaments into the surrounding tissue, tendons usually reattach themselves within a few days to a couple of weeks.

The best way to prevent recurrences after it has healed is to stretch the tendon daily.

Ruptured Achilles Tendon

In sports that require running, the Achilles tendon is subjected to more force and is ruptured far more commonly than any other tendon in the body. Ruptures of other tendons are rare and are usually the result of an unnatural force, as, for example, when a weight lifter lets a weight slip and it accidently tears a tendon in his wrist.

A tendon rupture becomes a serious medical problem either when the tendon recoils so far away from its original site that it can't reattach or when a piece of the bone is torn off with the tendon. In both of these conditions, it may be necessary to tie the tendon back in place with surgery.

Tendonitis

Causes

Tendonitis, an inflammation of the tendon which causes the tendon fibers to swell, is caused by tight muscles — the pulling at the tendon even when it is not being exercised.

Tendonitis is unique in that the pain is more intense when you first rise in the morning and lessens as you use the tendon. When you start a workout, your tendons will be extremely painful, and as you continue, the pain abates.

Dr. Don O'Donoghue, the dean of sportsmedicine physicians in America, says, "Tendonitis is one of the worst recurring problems in sportsmedicine. Because the pain decreases with exercise, the athlete won't stop exercising. He goes right back to performing the same thing that caused the problem in the first place."

Each sport has its most common site for tendonitis. In running sports — basketball, soccer, football, and track — it's Achilles tendonitis; in swimming and baseball, it's shoulder tendonitis; in tennis, it's elbow tendonitis.

Treatment

The treatment for all tendonitis is the same. When you first develop a pain in your tendon, stop all fast and hard exercise until the pain disappears. If you're a runner, just jog slowly. If the pain is severe when you jog, ride a bike. If you're a swimmer, use easy strokes that don't hurt. If you can't find a stroke that doesn't hurt, do kicking exercises in the water and hold on to a board. It may hurt less to try your stroke on an isokinetic machine, used by competitive swimmers to increase their strength.

A few days later when the pain is not so severe, you can try the only successful treatment for tendonitis — stretching. Remember, the cause of the damage to the tendon fiber is muscle tightness caused by hard exercise. When you stretch, do it slowly and gently, and hold your position for thirty seconds or longer. Quick, jerky stretches usually cause further damage to the tendon.

Do *not* ask your physician for steroid injections to alleviate the pain unless you are willing to stop exercising. They will only mask the pain, which will allow you to continue exercising and predispose you to further injury. Furthermore, there is medical evidence that steroid injections into a tendon will weaken it and make it more susceptible to tearing, if you continue to exercise. (See page 176.)

Bob McAdoo, basketball star with the New York Knicks, developed Achilles tendonitis. After the acute pain subsides, most professional players, including McAdoo, treat this injury by stretching.

"To stretch this tendon, McAdoo stands on an inclined board for twenty minutes before practices and games," reports Ray Melchiorre, his former trainer. "When the star of a team does something, so do the other players. Before long, the entire team lined up to stand on the board. Of course, now we don't have any Achilles tendon problems on the team."

The Two Ways to Stretch Your Achilles Tendon

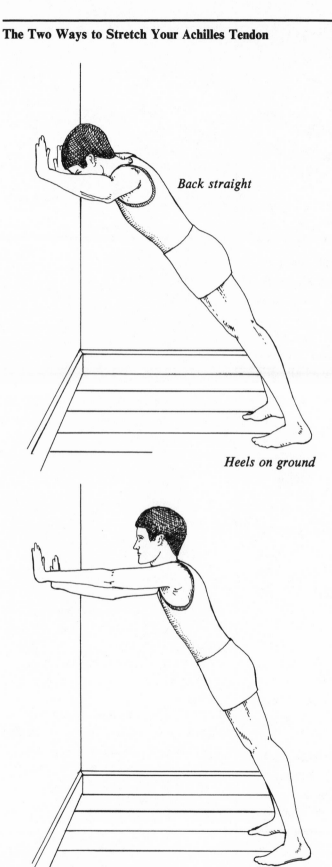

Back straight

Heels on ground

1. WALL PUSH-UPS

Standing at least four feet away, face a wall. Place your palms on the wall, keeping your back straight. Bend your elbows so your upper body will move closer to the wall. If you keep your heels on the ground, the calves and Achilles tendons will be stretched. Hold this position to the count of ten. Release the tension on your Achilles tendon by straightening your elbows and pushing your body away from the wall. Then repeat at least five times.

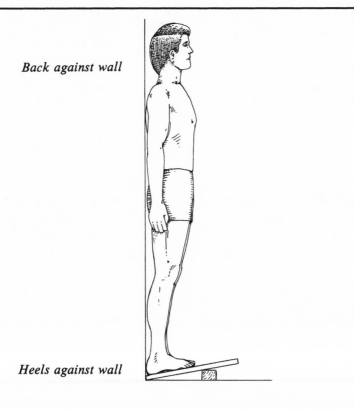

Back against wall

Heels against wall

2. BOARD STANDS

Place a board at least one foot long by one foot wide on the floor, with one end against the wall. Put any solid material two inches thick under the part of the board that is not against the wall. With your back and heels touching the wall, stand on the board for twenty to thirty minutes. To avoid boredom, read a book or watch television.

After a week or two, your tendon will be stretched and you can raise the height to four inches off the floor so the board is inclined even further. As your tendon becomes more flexible, you will be able to put a book under the stud and progressively increase the incline.

Because you lose your flexibility within a short time, you should stretch daily.

Bones

Your body has 208 bones, rigid and calcified structures that make up the skeleton, the framework of your body. Bones also serve as levers for muscles, protect the inner parts of your body, contain marrow which is the manufacturing plant for red blood cells, and are the storehouses for calcium and phosphorus.

If enough force is applied to any bone, it will break. A jarring tackle, a fall on the pavement, or repeated hard foot-strikes can cause breakage.

A break along the surface of the bone is called a fracture. There are two types of fractures:

A complete fracture, where the bone is severed completely
A stress fracture, where the bone is cracked, but not separated

Complete Fractures

Complete fractures are usually the most painful of all athletic injuries. The jagged edges of the separated bones

Complete Fracture

A complete fracture is a break in a bone that separates the ends.

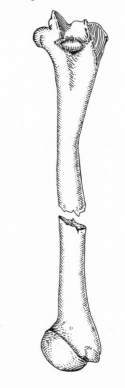

contain a rich supply of nerves and when they rub against each other or any other tissues, they cause extreme pain. The pain and swelling can continue for weeks or months. For that reason, many physicians routinely administer pain medicine to patients who have complete fractures.

Complete fractures require expert medical treatment. The sharp edges of a broken bone can cut a nerve and leave you paralyzed, can sever a blood vessel and cause you to bleed, and can cut through the skin and open a portal of entry for germs.

While some complete fractures of the small bones of the hands and feet heal by themselves, those of the large bones of the arms and legs often do not and should be checked immediately by an orthopedist. He will line up the bones properly so that they can heal without complications. This often requires taping, splinting, casting, or traction.

Complete breaks can take one to six months to heal, depending on the extent of the fracture, the treatment, and the absence of complications.

The Most Common Site for a Stress Fracture

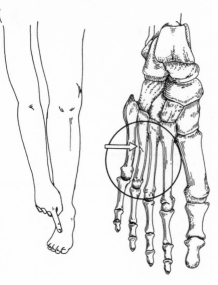

Stress Fractures

Causes

Stress fractures are slight cracks in the surface of the bones. The most common sites are the bones of the feet, legs, and hands.

I've had several stress fractures of my feet. They were the most painful injuries I've ever had.

Several years ago while running, I developed a slight pain in my foot which increased as I continued to run. When I stopped, the pain disappeared. The next day, as soon as I started to run, the pain recurred. Because I was training for the Boston Marathon, I tried to run through the pain but it was impossible. The farther I ran, the more it hurt. Finally, in spite of my bullheaded determination, my agony was so great that I had to stop. By then, I had extended the crack and for two weeks it ached all the time. After that, it hurt only to walk on it. It was the only injury that made me cry when I ran.

I believe that my stress fractures were due to my high-arched feet. This caused much of the force of my footstrike to be concentrated on the bones of my feet. It is the concentrated force on the bones that cracks them. Now that I cushion my footstrike with a soft support under my arch and wear track shoes with well-padded, thick soles, I

Athletes Who Suffered with Stress Fractures

Remarkably, 265-pound Carl Barzeloskus played his entire senior year at the University of Indiana with a stress fracture of his foot. His ability to handle the pain so impressed the scouts for the New York Jets that they drafted him number 1.

Marathoner Frank Shorter missed twenty-eight days of training because of a stress fracture. "In the last seven years, I've missed only seven days from everything else," says the famous runner. "My dad, who is a physician, put my foot in a cast because he knew it was the only way to stop me from running." His father used the cast to force Frank to accept the only successful treatment for stress fractures — rest. Usually four to fifteen weeks are required. The cast itself didn't aid the healing, because the bone was not actually separated.

don't break bones in my feet anymore. (See "High-Arched Feet," in Chapter 11.)

Diagnosis and treatment

How can you tell that you have a stress fracture? Use the finger test. A stress fracture usually hurts when you press on it with your finger both from above and below. A tendon or ligament usually hurts only on pressure from one side.

X rays usually are not sensitive enough to pick up small cracks in bones. It is not until two or three weeks later, when a callus — a layer of bony material — forms over the crack, that an X-ray diagnosis of a stress fracture can be made. By this time, if you have rested the fracture, the pain should have abated.

If you have a stress fracture, rest it and temporarily switch to another sport that will not extend the crack. For example, runners who develop stress fractures in their feet often change to riding a bicycle or swimming.

A sportsmedicine physician usually will not apply a cast to the injured area. Stress fractures heal by themselves in most cases. The immobilization caused by the cast makes the muscles smaller and weaker.

Bone Bruises

Sometimes the application of a sudden force to a bone, such as occurs when you step on a stone or bang your leg, can cause bone bruises, a bleeding under the outside covering of the bone. Although they may be painful, they usually heal within a few days and don't require any treatment or layoff from exercise. However, if you have a pain in your bone and it becomes worse with exercise, see your physician.

Joints and Cartilages

A joint is the place between two bones which functions like a hinge so that the bones can move in relation to each other. Cartilage, a tough white gristle that contains no blood vessels or nerves, lines the ends of the bones in a joint and protects them from rubbing against each other. If a cartilage is broken or chipped, the end of the unprotected

Diagram of a Joint

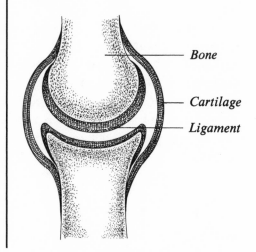

Bone

Cartilage

Ligament

bone can gradually wear down from friction against the cartilage of the opposing bone. Each movement will be painful because the end of the unprotected bone contains a rich supply of nerves.

Ligaments

Ligaments are tough fibrous bands that are attached near the ends of the bones as they meet to form the joint. Their main function is to hold the bones together when the joint moves.

Ligaments can hold the bones together so tightly that there is very little movement of the joint. For example, the vertebrae in your spine, held together by ligaments, can move only slightly. Ligaments can also be flexible enough to allow a wide range of motion. Good examples of mobile joints are those of the extremities — the wrist, elbow, shoulder, ankle, knee, and hip.

If some of the fibers of the ligament are torn, it is called a sprain. To avoid further tearing of these fibers, the joint should be immobilized immediately. If all of the fibers are torn, the injury is called a complete ligamentous rupture. In most cases, the ligament reattaches itself by laying down new cells, but sometimes surgery will be necessary.

All joint injuries, whether they involve bones, cartilage, ligaments, or the muscles and tendons that attach near the joint, have the potential to end your athletic career.

If you incur an injury to a joint, whether it is your ankle, knee, hip, wrist, elbow, or shoulder, treat it immediately with RICE. Never exercise a joint that has just been injured. If the pain or swelling is severe or lasts beyond twenty-four hours, seek help from a sportsmedicine physician.

I realize that, in most cases, the pain will not be gone in twenty-four hours, and as a result many people will be checking with their physicians needlessly. However, the diagnosis and management of joint injuries require expertise that cannot be taught in a book. Therefore, I would rather send you to a physician needlessly than take the chance that you will not receive adequate treatment for a potentially serious problem.

Surgical Success Stories

Pat Stapleton of the Chicago Black Hawks slammed into a goal post at 25 miles an hour, destroying his knee cartilages. One doctor immediately put the injured leg in a cast. When the cast was removed six weeks later, Stapleton's knee was frozen in a bent position. He couldn't move it at all and there was some question whether Stapleton would ever walk again. Another physician, Ted Fox, was consulted.

"Dr. Fox told me to prop up Stapleton's leg on a chair and sit on it," recalls Skip Thayer, the Black Hawk trainer. "After I had sat on Pat's knee for several weeks, the leg began to straighten and Dr. Fox operated. It's a medical miracle that Pat was able to play hockey again."

Another remarkable surgical success story we found is the case of Emerson Boozer of the New York Jets.

As a rookie in 1966, he scored thirteen touchdowns in six games and was on his way to break Gale Sayers's touchdown record. In a game against Kansas City, he made a great catch and was tackled both high and low while turning. He was hit with such force that every structure in his knee was damaged: his ligaments were torn; his cartilage was fractured; his kneecap was dislocated; and even part of his thigh muscle was torn.

"I flew back to New York City with him and operated on him at midnight," recalls Dr. James Nicholas, the team physician. In essence, Dr. Nicholas had to rebuild the entire knee, and, as a result, Boozer was able to continue playing professional football for ten more years.

Tennis queen Billy Jean King also had successful knee surgery. One major reason for her excellent rehabilitation: a comprehensive exercise program to strengthen the muscles that support her knee.

Knee Injuries

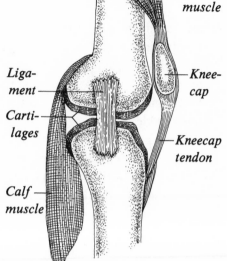

The most famous joint in sports is the knee.

"You tell a professional athlete that he has a knee injury and he immediately thinks his career is finished," says Dr. James Nicholas. "Some athletes start crying."

Gale Sayers, Dick Butkus, Larry Brown, and Joe Namath, four outstanding National Football League players, had their careers cut short by knee injuries. Bobby Orr, once considered the greatest star in hockey, underwent many knee operations, and was forced to retire at a very early age.

Why are knee injuries so common?

"The knee is not a very stable joint," explains Dr. Don O'Donoghue, who specializes in knee operations. "It's just two long bones held together by ligaments."

Football, hockey, basketball, and soccer players are particularly likely to suffer such injuries because of the physical contact.

Hockey player Derek Sanderson explains why players of that sport are so susceptible: "Once you make a cut, your body is committed to where your feet go. It's impossible to get your foot out of that rut. If you come in contact with another body going twenty-five miles an hour, your knee is automatically going to go. You'll tear all the ligaments and cartilages in the knee."

There are at least five places where the knee can be injured: the cartilages, the ligaments, the muscles around the knees, the kneecap (a bone in front of the joint), and the kneecap tendons. If you sustain a knee injury, see an orthopedist immediately.

How to guard against knee injuries

If you participate in contact sports such as football, there are four good ways to help protect yourself against knee injuries:

Don't wear cleats. They anchor your foot to the ground. Many pro teams now use cleatless shoes.

Run with short, choppy steps. The less time the foot is on the ground, the less likelihood of knee injury. If you anticipate being hit, shorten your stride.

If possible, protect your knees from a hit, especially from the back and side. That's where the knee is most susceptible to injury and is one reason the National Football League outlawed crackback blocks.

Exercise the muscles around the knee. There's evidence that these exercises thicken ligaments and make them more resistant to injury.

Sprained Ligaments

A sprained ligament is a partial or complete rupture of the ligaments that hold the joints together. Basketball and football players get sprains in the ankle and knee, tennis players in the elbow, high jumpers in the knee, and bowlers in the thumb. The most common form of this injury is a sprained ankle.

When you develop a pain in your ankle, knee, hip, wrist, elbow, or shoulder, stop exercising. If the pain persists, treat the injury in the same manner that you would treat a muscle pull: with RICE. If you think the injury is severe, or if you have swelling, see a sportsmedicine physician. I caution you that ligaments are part of a joint and all joint injuries can be serious. You may have a fractured bone or a torn ligament or muscle.

Exercise will strengthen ligaments and render them less susceptible to injury. When I first started to run, I sprained my ankle several times. It took a while before I realized the cause. Because I was running in open fields — full of potholes and depressions — I was turning my ankles slightly with each step. However, as I continued to run, the severity of my sprains decreased and finally after six months, my problem went away completely. My running program had thickened my ligaments and tendons and made them far more resistant to injuries.

People who repeatedly sprain their ankles often have pronated or flat feet. Pronation can be treated with high-top sneakers or special shoes with arch supports. (See "Excessive Pronation of the Feet," in Chapter 11.)

Low-Back Pain

Low-back pain is usually the result of excess stretching of the ligaments of the spine. In athletes the two most common causes are:

A muscle imbalance in which the curvature of the lower back is increased. This is called lumbar lordosis and is correctable with exercise.

Doug Collins of the Philadelphia 76ers sprained his ankle several times in the 1976–77 season.

"We have a special machine that wraps and cools the injured ankle," says Gary Gordon, the team podiatrist. "With this procedure we got Collins to play the night after he sprained it."

A Daily Exercise to Strengthen the Muscles around the Knee

LEG EXTENSIONS

1. Attach a 5-pound weight to your shoes or feet. These weights usually cost about $20 in any sports store.
2. Sit in a chair with your knees bent.
3. Slowly raise your foot to the level pictured in the diagram.
4. Hold the top position for 1 second.
5. Repeat ten times. Rest for 30 seconds. Then do four more sets of ten. Rest between each set.
6. Repeat with other foot.

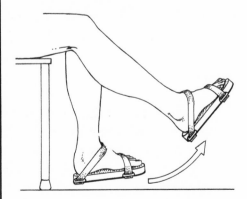

The best way to strengthen the muscles around your knee is to run in snow or sand, when available.

A forward slippage of one of the segments of the spine, commonly called a slipped disk. If the pain in your back is severe or radiates down the back of your leg, you might have this potentially serious medical condition and you should be checked by a physician.

When you were in grade school, your teacher probably put one hand on your back and the other on your belly and then gave you a grade for posture. If you had a minimal curve in your lower back, you received an A. If you had a deep curve, you received a D. An exaggerated curvature of your lower back stretches the ligaments that hold the vertebrae together and can cause pain.

The curvature of your lower back is determined by the tilt of your pelvis. If your pelvis is tilted backward, the curve decreases.

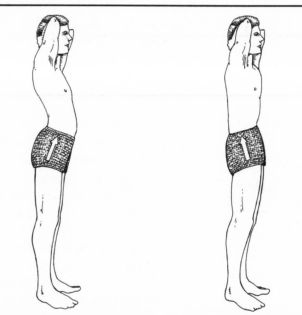

Pelvis tilted forward causing an exaggerated curvature of the back   *Normal back curvature*

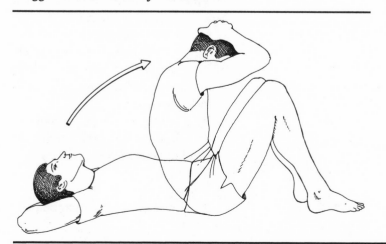

Bent-Knee Sit-ups

(Because exercise can aggravate certain types of disk problems in the spine, check with your physician before doing this exercise.)

The best way to shorten your abdominal muscles is to perform bent-knee sit-ups with weights.

Start with three sets of ten bent-knee sit-ups without weights. After you become proficient, start using weights. I recommend that you wrap a 2½-pound weight in a towel and hold it behind your head. Do three sets of ten sit-ups. As you become stronger, increase the weight. You will develop adequate abdominal muscles faster by increasing the weights than by increasing the number of sit-ups.

Straight-legged sit-ups don't develop abdominal muscles. They tighten a muscle called the iliopsoas that runs from the pelvis to the inner side of the thigh bones. When this muscle is tightened, it actually increases the curve in your back, the structural abnormality that you are trying to correct.

Low-back pain is far more common in women than men. High heels and pregnancy shift their weight forward and increase the curve in the back, causing low-back pain. Potbellied men also have their weight shifted forward and often have low-back pain.

If you suddenly develop a pain in your back, rest. If after a few days the pain continues, see a physician.

Many cases of low-back pain can be treated with stretching and strengthening exercises. To decrease the curve in your back, you should tilt your pelvis forward. To do this, you must perform exercises that shorten your abdominal muscles and stretch the muscles in your back.

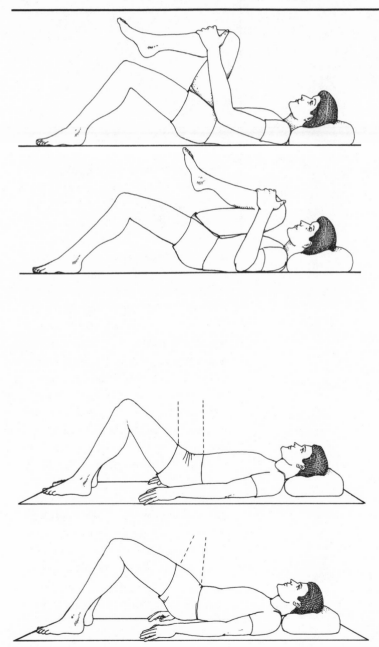

The Low-Back Stretch

To stretch the muscles in your back, do the four stretching exercises — the plow, the Japanese split, the toe touch and the wall push-up — described on page 140 in Chapter 11. If your back hurts, do not perform the plow. In its place, substitute the following low-back stretch.

1. Lie on your back with a pillow under your head and bend your knees.
2. As shown in the diagram, place your hands on your right leg.
3. With your hands, pull your knee to your chest and hold for 10 seconds.
4. Lower the leg to the floor.
5. Repeat with the other leg.
6. Perform this exercise twenty-five times with each leg.

To help you decrease the curve in your back, I recommend the pelvic tilt.
1. Lie on your back with a pillow under your head and bend your knees.
2. Press the small of your back toward the ground and squeeze your buttocks together.
3. By putting your weight on your shoulders and heels and keeping the small of your back flat, raise your hips a few inches.
4. Hold this position for 10 seconds.
5. Relax and repeat this exercise ten times.

Fascia

Faceiae are the strong thick white fibrous sheets that surround, protect, and support almost all the tissue in the body: muscles, tendons, joints, nerves, blood vessels, and organs. Fascia looks and feels to some degree like ligaments and tendons and contains the same four components: two types of fibers, fluid, and connective tissue cells.

In athletes, fasciae absorb some of the pressure on tendons, muscles, and joints, and help protect them from injury.

Plantar Fasciitis

The most common athletic injury to the fascia is called plantar fasciitis, a partial or complete tear of the fascia that covers the muscles on the bottom of the feet. It is usually characterized by pain just under the heel bone, but the pain can also occur anywhere on the bottom of the foot. The pain can start immediately with a sudden tear during exercise or can develop gradually over many days. There is usually no swelling.

The plantar fascia extends from the bottom part of the heel bone to each of the five toes. It serves as a guide wire to support the bottom of the foot, especially the arch. If sufficient pressure is exerted on the bottom of your foot — enough to spread out the toes or to flatten the arch — the fascia tears. Here are four main causes of plantar fasciitis:

1. A sudden turn that exerts great pressure on the tissues on the bottom of the foot. According to Frank Challant, the trainer for the former world-champion Boston Celtics: "Just before the 1975 playoffs, John Havlicek zigged when he should have zagged. The sudden force tore his plantar fascia and we rested him through the entire series against Buffalo. Then I used a special taping procedure that supported his arch and took pressure off the plantar fascia. He was able to play and helped the Celtics beat Cleveland and Phoenix for the World Championship."

2. Shoes that don't have adequate support for the arch of the foot. Running back John Riggins of the Washington Redskins developed his fasciitis from wearing shoes with too much flexibility and not enough support. According to Dr. James Nicholas, "Riggins was wearing a ballet-type slipper on the Astroturf in the Orange Bowl. We treated

Location of Plantar Fasciitis

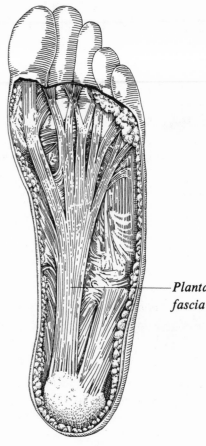

Plantar fascia

his injury with special shoes that had special supports for his arch."

3. Shoes that have very stiff soles. Every week I see several runners who have plantar fasciitis caused by track shoes with very stiff soles. Every time you run, you land on your heel and step off on your toes. If the sole is very stiff, you have to use extra force to bend it. This extra force is concentrated on the plantar fascia and can tear it. Flexible-soled shoes and arch supports are the best treatment.

4. Feet that pronate excessively. People whose feet pronate excessively — that is, their feet roll inward when they walk or run — are more likely to develop plantar fasciitis. By dropping the arch and spreading out the toes, pronation puts added tension on the plantar fascia. In this case, the treatment is orthotics. (See "Excessive Pronation of the Feet," in Chapter 11.)

A few years ago a leading middle-distance runner got plantar fasciitis from running fast intervals. Because he was preparing for the upcoming Olympics, he couldn't rest. Instead, he received anti-inflammatory steroid injections (cortisone), which decreased the pain. These shots do not promote healing. The athlete's foot did not heal in time and, sadly, he missed the Olympics.

I do not believe that steroid injections should be used to treat plantar fasciitis. Not only can they weaken the fascia, but also they can stop the pain — nature's warning signal that you should be taking it easy — and by continuing to exercise, you cause further damage.

Heel Spur

Heel Spurs

Some surgeons feel that a heel spur, a small, extra piece of heel bone that sticks out where the plantar fascia attaches, causes some cases of plantar fasciitis. But many people have heel spurs and don't have foot pain. Some orthopedists operate on painful heel spurs to treat plantar fasciitis, but most orthopedists feel they are best left alone.

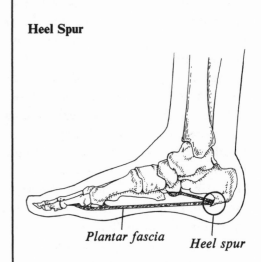

Plantar fascia   *Heel spur*

Summary: Long-Term Treatment for Injuries to the Six Internal Tissues and Structures

Muscles are treated with strengthening exercises.

Tendons are treated with stretching exercises.

Bones usually heal themselves, after a physician has aligned them so that they will knit together properly.

Joint therapy is complex and should be given by a sportsmedicine physician.

Ligament injuries can be severe and should usually be treated by a physician.

Fascial injuries of the feet are treated with mechanical supports or taping to relieve the pressure that originally caused the injury. Surgery may be required for some fascial injuries.

Skin

The skin is the outermost covering of your body and consequently is at high risk of being damaged, injured, and infected. It is remarkable how well the skin stands up to the continual onslaught of germs, dirt, pollutants, scrapes, bangs, friction, sun, wind, heat, and cold. Your skin lasts as long as you live, which is many times the usual lifetime of other surface coverings, such as paint or clothes. There are reasons your skin lasts so long and so well:

It is constantly replacing itself with new cells. You grow a new surface layer of skin every twenty-eight days. If you cut yourself, the skin will grow up to seven times faster to repair itself.

It is specially adapted in many ways to resist damage. For example, it tends to maintain a dry outer surface, which prevents germs (which require water) from surviving or growing. Wetness provides an environment that frequently leads to infection.

It can respond to protect itself. For example, if skin is frequently and vigorously rubbed, as occurs in many sports, it will protect itself by forming a thick covering called a callus.

Skin injuries often result when there are predisposing functional or structural abnormalities. For example, an athlete who does not tan easily and cannot form a protective layer of pigment is more likely to sunburn when he is exposed to the noonday sun. An exerciser whose fourth and fifth toes are particularly close together, thus preventing perspiration from evaporating from between these toes, is predisposed to infection at this site, i.e., athlete's foot.

In many cases, skin injuries, like injuries to other tissues, can be prevented by correcting or compensating for the predisposing factors.

Abrasions

An abrasion is an injury in which some of the skin is scraped off through some unusual or abnormal mechanical process. It is frequently the result of falling onto a hard, rough, or jagged surface. Cyclists get abrasions from falling on the pavement. Football players get them from falling on artificial turf, and boxers can get them when they are hit.

Rarely are abrasions deep enough to cause any serious problems. You usually don't develop a scar unless the wound cuts right through to the deeper layers of skin.

What do you do when you suffer an abrasion? The most important part of treatment is to remove all foreign material from the wound, such as dirt or glass. Run hydrogen peroxide or water over the area to wash it thoroughly.

A wound may be too painful or too deep in the skin to wash thoroughly. In that case, see a physician. He will inject an anesthetic near the edges of the wound so it can be cleaned thoroughly without discomfort. He may also give you an antibiotic to kill germs and, in the case of a deep wound, a tetanus shot.

Don't apply alcohol to an abrasion because it will irritate your skin. Instead, apply an antibiotic ointment, such as Mycitracin, Neo-Polycin, Neosporin, or Polysporin, which you can buy in a drugstore without a prescription.

If possible, don't cover a wound. A tight covering keeps the area moist and predisposes to growth of bacteria. To prevent your clothes from rubbing on the wound and dirt from getting into it, you may need to apply a light gauze pad loosely over the antibiotic ointment. However, remove the pad each night to let the wound dry out.

Healing time depends on several factors, including your age and the location of the wound. Children heal much faster than older people. Also, a small wound of the face will heal in three days while the same size wound on the leg may take more than a week. The reason: The face has a better blood supply, which carries nutrients to the wound and promotes healing.

There are several things you can do to prevent abrasions.

Always wear protective equipment when participating in sports in which falls or body contact are common. Take measures when possible to improve the type and condition of the playing field.

Blisters

Blisters are localized collections of fluid in the outer part of the skin. In athletes and fitness enthusiasts, they are usually the result of persistent or repeated rubbing against the skin. Pitchers get them on their pitching hand from gripping the baseball. Runners get them on the soles of their feet from running in loose shoes. Bicycle racers get them on their behinds from rubbing against the seat.

To protect your feet from blisters, the shoe must fit like a glove. Thick socks prevent a glovelike fit. More than one-third of the National Hockey League players, including Bobby Orr and Wayne Cashman, don't wear socks at all. Most marathon runners, including Frank Shorter, often shun socks. The only reason to wear socks is to prevent odor.

Some marathoners and Ray Melchiorre of the Buffalo Braves prevent foot blisters by covering their feet with Vaseline. If you are prone to blistering, try rubbing Vaseline into the shoe at sites where it rubs against your skin.

Another trick is to put plain adhesive tape (with no gauze) over the blister site. The shoe will rub against the tape instead of against your skin.

Studies by U.S. Army doctors have shown that blisters heal faster when the fluid is drained. First, cleanse the blister site with alcohol. Then sterilize a needle by heating it over a flame until it turns red. After allowing the needle to cool, use it to puncture the blister at its edge and drain the fluid by pressing on the top of the blister. Do *not* remove the skin over the blister because you will be creating an open wound which is far more susceptible to infection.

Then take plain adhesive tape (with no gauze) and apply it tightly over the blister. Most of the time, you can resume exercising immediately. Leave the tape in place until it comes off by itself.

The only side effect I have ever seen from this procedure is infection and it is extremely rare. If the area becomes

Carmen Salvino says the most common injury to professional bowlers is a blister on the bowling thumb. "Don't laugh, it can destroy your game."

quite painful, oozes pus, or develops red streaks, see a physician immediately.

Blisters can often be prevented if you wear proper-fitting and adequate sports equipment. For example, blister formation can be reduced by regular use of a golf glove, particularly in the early part of the season before the hand has formed protective calluses.

Athlete's Foot

Athlete's foot is a term that refers to two different conditions of the toes and soles of the feet. One, caused by a fungus (ringworm), is usually dry, scaly, and itchy; the other, caused by bacteria, is usually wet, malodorous, and painful.

Fungus infections may be picked up by walking barefoot around a pool or in a shower room. They usually develop between the fourth and fifth toes, which are the closest together, or on the sole in cases where feet perspire in hot, tight shoes. Mold fungus infections often respond to Tolnaftate, a nonprescription medication, and clear up within one to two weeks. More severe cases require special prescription medications from your physician.

The bacterial form of athlete's foot commonly follows a fungus infection and when it occurs, fungus medications are useless. Treatment consists of separation of the toes, drying lotions, and oral antibiotics. With proper treatment, it improves in a couple of days and may be cured in a week. See a dermatologist to obtain the proper medications.

Both types of athlete's foot occur when the feet become very wet — from exercise, tight shoes, hot weather, and perspiration. Keeping the feet dry by exposing them to air or sprinkling them with powder is often helpful in preventing such flareups. Showering and thorough drying of the feet as well as changing socks after your feet have perspired are basic rules that should always be followed after athletic activity.

If your feet tend to perspire excessively, see a dermatologist. He will give you special medications to control this condition.

"Jock Itch"

"Jock itch" is a red, flaky rash that develops in the groin and upper, inner parts of the thighs. It is usually due to a fungus infection but can also be caused by yeast or bacteria, particularly in more severe cases. As in cases of athlete's foot, warm weather, excessive sweating, and prolonged wearing of wet underclothes are predisposing factors.

If you develop a mild groin rash that is ring-shaped or has a sharp border, go to a drugstore and buy a skin cream that will kill fungi. As several preparations are highly irritating, I recommend Tolnaftate. It should heal in one to two weeks. If the condition persists or becomes more severe, or if the rash looks different from that just described, see a dermatologist. By examining you, checking for diseases that can cause "jock itch," looking at skin scrapings under a microscope, and doing diagnostic cultures, he will be able to determine the cause and institute effective treatment.

Dr. Ronald Shore, my associate, once treated a professional golfer for a severe case of "jock itch" just after the golfer had won a national tournament. The rash had apparently resulted from excessive perspiration and had become badly infected with bacteria. The public never knew that by the day the tournament ended, the rash had become so severe that the golfer couldn't even sit down! The rash was treated with antibiotics and a drying agent, and quickly resolved.

Plantar Warts

Plantar warts are warts that have developed on the sole of the foot. Warts are rough spots that to some degree resemble calluses. Unlike calluses, however, they do not show the normal fingerprintlike patterns of the skin surface.

Warts are caused by a particular type of virus germ that can invade the top layer of skin. Plantar warts are commonly contracted when you walk barefoot where somebody with plantar warts has previously passed. If you suspect that you have them, see a dermatologist immediately because they can multiply and spread to others. They frequently do not go away by themselves and often are so painful that you end up walking or running unnaturally and suffer further injury. I usually remove them surgically.

Sunburn

Today, with increased interest in sports and exercise, people are out of doors in greater numbers for longer periods. As a result, physicians are seeing more cases of sun-induced injuries than ever before.

A single exposure to sunlight can cause sunburn. The severity of sunburn ranges from slight redness of the skin with a feeling of warmth, to deep painful blisters. The initial redness and swelling are due to a widening of the blood vessels in the skin with a leakage of fluid into the surrounding tissue. The body responds in the same way it would to a blow. The only difference is that in sunburn, redness usually appears more slowly — in two to six hours, reaching its maximum intensity in twelve to twenty-four hours.

The redness from a sunburn can last from several hours to several days and is often followed by a peeling of the superficial skin. If the burn is mild, redness is the only reaction. However, if the burn is more severe, deep blisters followed by scabbing and even scarring can result.

There are two chief factors which determine how much damage, if any, a person will incur from sun exposure.

The amount of protective pigment in the person's skin at the time of exposure

People vary tremendously in their susceptibility to sun damage. Blacks and other dark-complexioned individuals have skin which is capable of producing large amounts of pigment, and consequently are far less susceptible to the ravages of sunlight. But skin pigment does not block sunlight completely, and with very prolonged and extremely intense exposure even darkly pigmented skin can be damaged. The fairer your skin, the more susceptible you are to all the previously mentioned forms of sun damage. If your skin tends to tan poorly, you must be especially careful in protecting it.

When your eyes are exposed to bright sun, the retina (the membrane at the back of the eye which transmits the images to the brain) can also be burned. To protect your eyes when you're out in the bright sun, wear sunglasses. They screen out the harmful rays of the sun that can damage your eyes.

The amount and intensity of sunlight

Sunlight is most intense when the sun is directly overhead, because fewer rays are screened out by the atmosphere. This occurs during the summer, particularly between 10:00 A.M. and 2:00 P.M. (or between 11:00 A.M. and 3:00 P.M. if you are on Daylight Savings Time). If you are prone to sun damage, avoid training or competing during this time of day or take other precautions.

The skin can be damaged even on hazy days because 50 percent of the rays that reach your skin are rays that are reflected off clouds, the ground or a house — not coming directly from the sun.

Snow reflects over 85 percent of the sun's burning rays. Consequently, skiers can be burned in the wintertime. It has recently been shown that wind can intensify sun damage, which explains why downhill skiers are particularly prone to sunburn. Sand also reflects considerable light, so persons on a beach can suffer sun damage even if under an umbrella. Water can also reflect the sun's rays, so people who participate in water sports must also protect themselves.

Several drugs, foods, and lotions can make your skin burn, itch, and swell when it is exposed to an amount of sunlight that normally wouldn't bother you at all. If you suddenly develop an irritation from sunlight, check the list in the accompanying sidebar.

How to Avoid Sunburn

If you are fair-skinned, or if you are exposed to the intense sun of the tropics or the reflected sun from sand, snow, or water, here are some simple rules to follow:

Avoid the sun between 10:00 A.M. and 2:00 P.M. That's when the sun's rays are most intense.

Wear clothing that protects your skin from the sun. I recommend a wide-brimmed hat. Don't wear porous clothing, because the sun's rays will pass through to your skin. Even most men's white shirts permit 20 percent of the sun's burning rays to reach the skin. Some blouses worn by women may transmit more than 50 percent of the rays. White is the preferred color because it reflects the sun's rays.

Acquire a tan gradually. Gradual exposure to the sun increases the pigment in your skin, which blocks much of the harmful effects of the sun's rays.

Use lotions to block or screen out the sun's rays. There are several types of chemicals in commercial sun lotions: ones that *screen out* the damaging rays but let some tanning rays through, such as PABA; and ones that *block* all the sun's rays so that even tanning is prevented, such as zinc oxide.

Drugs and Chemicals That May Make Your Skin More Susceptible to Sun Damage

ANTIBIOTICS	Nalidixic acid
	Sulfa drugs
	Tetracyclines
ANTIFUNGAL AGENTS	Griseofulvin
ANTIHISTAMINES	Diphenhydramine
ARTIFICIAL SWEETENERS	Saccharin
	Sodium cyclohexyl-sulfamate
	Sucaryl
COAL TAR DERIVATIVES	Over-the-counter ointments
DIABETES MEDICATIONS	Chlorpropamide
	Tolbutamide
DIURETICS	Chlorothiazide
	Hydrochlorothiazide
DYES	Acridine
	Eosin
	Methylene blue
HEART MEDICATIONS	Quinidine
PLANT OILS	Oil of bergamot
	Oil of cedar
	Oil of citron
	Oil of lavender
PSORIASIS MEDICATIONS	Coal tar
	Psoralen
SUNSCREENS	PABA and PABA derivatives*
TRANQUILIZERS	Chlorpromazine
	Chlorprothezine
	Mepazine
	Perpheniazine
	Prochlorperazine
	Promethazine
	Triflupromazine

*Paradoxically, sunscreens containing PABA and, more commonly, certain PABA derivatives, sometimes actually increase one's reaction to sunlight.

One of the most effective lotions, a commercial ointment called RVPaque, contains both PABA and zinc oxide. It blocks out the sun's rays completely and doesn't wash off easily when you exercise. But many people do not like to use it because they find it greasy and they usually want to acquire some tan.

PABA without zinc oxide in a lotion or gel form is an acceptable alternative. But it is only a sunscreen. In my opinion, Pre-Sun, Sundown, and Sungard are excellent sunscreens. Certain PABA derivatives (glyceryl PABA, sometimes called Escalol 106, and Padimate A — they will be on the label of the sun lotion) often cause skin rashes, according to new studies by Dr. Alexander Fisher of New York University and Dr. Albert Kligman of the University of Pennsylvania, both famous professors of dermatology.

When you use these sunscreens, remember some can be easily removed by perspiration and as a result you must reapply them frequently, according to directions on the label. Cocoa butter and mineral oils are not effective sunscreens. If you use them when exposed to intense sunlight, your skin will simply be fried instead of broiled.

How to Treat Sunburn

Apply a soothing ointment and take two aspirin tablets every four hours for one day. Aspirin blocks the pain. Caution: The aspirin may upset your stomach. If you are allergic to aspirin or if the pain is severe, see your physician, who will probably prescribe some form of cortisone, the most effective and rapid medication for sunburn relief.

Recent studies have shown that a lotion containing indomethacin, a drug for the treatment of arthritis, is also effective in blocking the pain and inflammation.

There are several commercial, over-the-counter preparations that can be applied to sunburn. Many of these contain anesthetics or antihistamines and, in my opinion, should be avoided because they can cause allergic reactions.

Actinic Keratoses

After many years of exposure to sunlight, you may develop small scaly areas, called actinic keratoses, on your sun-damaged skin. They're common in light-skinned individuals over fifty years of age. Actinic keratoses are not serious in themselves but can become skin cancers if not treated. They can be removed by surgery, special chemicals, electric current, or liquid nitrogen freezing.

Skin Cancers

Skin cancers can develop from actinic keratoses or from normal-appearing skin. They are almost always the result of previous sun damage and appear on those parts of the body that are most exposed to sun, i.e., the forehead, the tops of the ears, cheeks, nose, and backs of the hands. Many skin cancers have depressed centers and raised pearl-colored borders covered by one or more tiny blood vessels. They can start out as small as the tip of a pin or grow to cover much of the face.

These slow-growing tumors usually do not spread to other parts of the body and thus rarely kill. However, they can cause considerable damage if neglected. They can be cured in almost all cases by various surgical procedures or radiation therapy. See a dermatologist if you think you have this condition.

11.

How to Avoid Injuries

Minor injuries can cause an athlete to miss training and competition. Major ones can end his or her career. Injuries have cost some teams championships while other teams have won them because they remain healthy. Even people who exercise for fitness in low-intensity sports have become injured, and injuries are the most common cause of exercisers dropping out of their fitness programs.

Many injuries are preventable. Here are some examples from my files and the files of other sportsmedicine physicians:

A New York Yankee superstar is forced into early retirement after surgery for a heel spur. A special shoe fitted with a custom insert might have saved him from that surgery. Unfortunately it wasn't available twenty years ago.

A national amateur tennis champion undergoes surgery for tennis elbow and never plays again. Special strengthening exercises should have been tried first.

A weight lifter develops sciatica — a sharp pain in the lower back that sometimes extends down the back of one or both legs. After six weeks of bed rest and three months with no training, he is no better. Corrective exercises to change the curve of his back cure him in six weeks.

A basketball player develops shin splints. Cortisone injections, taping, and ultrasound treatments fail to ease the pain. Stretching and strengthening exercises cure him in a few weeks.

An All-American lacrosse player pulls his hamstring muscle in three consecutive seasons. Taught to correct

Devastating Injuries

The 1976 U.S. Olympic team was decimated by injuries. Steve Williams and Houston McTear, two of the best sprinters in America, and Marty Liquori, the country's leading middle-distance runner, all pulled muscles and didn't even make the team.

Because of knee problems All-Pro football players Gale Sayers, Larry Brown, and Dick Butkus were forced into early retirement.

Sandy Koufax of the Los Angeles Dodgers, possibly the greatest pitcher of all time, retired because of a severe case of pitcher's elbow.

an imbalance between his hamstring and the muscle in front of his thigh, he reports no further problems.

An excellent college cross-country runner undergoes surgery for runner's knee and never runs again. The preferred treatment: use of special inserts, called orthotics, in his shoes.

A sixteen-year-old high school halfback submits to a third painful cortisonelike injection in the Achilles tendon. In his next scrimmage, he tears the tendon from his heel and is still limping a year later.

Once you are injured, your physician can do little to speed the healing process. He can close wounds and set broken bones so that they will heal more quickly. He can prevent and treat complications such as infection and prevent further extension of your injury. But in general, rest is the best treatment.

In the long run, it's important that you or your physician discover and correct the factors that caused your injury:

Overtraining, where you push beyond your limits

Poor training methods, where you increase the intensity or the amount of training too rapidly

A structural abnormality in your body that puts added stress on muscles, tendons, bones, joints, faciae, and ligaments

Lack of flexibility (muscles tightened by hard exercise are more susceptible to injury)

Muscle imbalance, where one muscle overpowers another that performs an opposite function

Even professional athletes, who have available to them the best treatments that physicians can offer, can lose time, seasons, and even their careers to an injury.

The Overtraining Syndrome

Far and away the most common cause of sports injuries stems from overwork. Do not be so intent on training that you ignore the warning signals sent out by your body. The most important signal: persistent pain in muscles, bones, or joints.

The uses of pain

In the fall of 1975, one of the premier runners in the world and I were speakers at a runner's clinic held in conjunction

An Injury That Never Happened

In 1975, with his right leg and left arm in casts and using crutches, Sparky Lyle, the first relief pitcher ever to win the Cy Young Award, reported to the spring training camp of the world-champion New York Yankees. He hobbled across the field to tell manager Bill Virdon that he had been in a terrible automobile accident and was through for the season.

It was very tense for several minutes," recalls a teammate. "Many of us could see the World Series slipping away."

It was all a hoax. Lyle, one of baseball's great practical jokers, had convinced a doctor friend to rig up the casts.

**Spending More to Protect
Their Investment**

In the last five years, some professional teams have doubled their spending on medical services. "To protect million-dollar athletes, every team invests more in medical care, especially for prevention," notes Dr. James Nicholas.

Ken Moore and Bob Scharf, two of the country's top marathoners during the 1960s, recently lectured on distance running to my class on sports-medicine at the University of Maryland.

Scharf told the students that he used to run more than 150 miles a week, and once won two marathons in six days. His career was marred by many injuries and operations.

Moore, a two-time Olympian, runs slightly more than half as much and is rarely injured.

— GABE MIRKIN, M.D.

with the National A.A.U. Cross Country Championship in Annapolis, Maryland.

In my presentation I said that a runner who develops localized tenderness that becomes worse as he or she runs should abandon a workout. I explained that pain is a body defense mechanism that warns that the body has a problem, such as torn muscle fibers, sprained ligaments, or internal muscle bleeding. I noted that failure to heed such signals can make the injury worse and prolong the healing time.

The champion runner, in his speech, argued that all runners get local tenderness and should not let it limit their workouts. He subsequently was injured — presumably while following his own advice — and was forced to miss the 1976 Olympics. His determination to endure pain helped him become a great runner, but it appears to have made him more susceptible to injury.

It should not surprise you that novices are injured far more frequently than top athletes. One difference is conditioning. Another is that experienced athletes understand that pain is nature's signal, warning them to stop. I've had recurring injuries over the years. Early in my career, I tried to run through pain. Now I'm much smarter. When I develop pain that increases as I run, I stop and go home.

People who are competitive are more likely to suffer from overtraining. It is this motivation that often drives them to ignore pain. I see overtraining not only in great athletes whose livelihood depends on their performances, but also in fitness buffs such as business executives on the squash courts and housewives in a Run For Your Life program.

Rest

Sometimes a professional athlete must go out on the field even though he knows that he shouldn't. That's how he earns his paycheck.

Larry Brown, the former Washington Redskin All-Pro running back, feels that most serious football injuries occur because the athlete plays before he has healed. "In the professional leagues," Brown says, "rest is like cursing in church. You got to be ready each Sunday."

John Riggins, the $300,000-a-year running back now with the Washington Redskins, refuses to play when hurt. Riggins feels that injuries must be given time to heal.

From a medical point of view, Riggins is right. Time is

Once, some players were lying around in the training room because they feared the practice or had minor injuries. Coach Vince Lombardi stalked in and gruffly asked, "What are these people doing in here? What's wrong with them?"

Suddenly everyone came to life. Crutches went flying and the players ran all over each other trying to get to the field. He cleared the whole training room."

— *Former All-Pro running back*
LARRY BROWN
of the Washington Redskins

The Real Professional

In the 1975 season, Joe Namath, then with the Jets, suffered from swollen knees.

"We gave Broadway Joe a three-gallon Gatorade container filled with ice," says Tim Davey, the Jet's assistant trainer. "He was told to ice down his knees all night. He never complained in public or said that he wouldn't play."

the best healer. When stress is applied to an injured tendon, muscle, or ligament, further injury usually results.

Training and overtraining

An athlete is limited by the number of hard workouts he can take in a given period of time. Jack Mahurin, a professor at Springfield College in Massachusetts and a top-flight marathon runner, says that the difference between a good runner and a great one is that a good one can run hard twice a week, while a great one can run hard three times a week. The purpose of training is to expose the body to repeated stress in the form of hard workouts or races. The art of training is to know how much hard work the body can handle before it breaks down or is injured.

The overtraining syndrome can be divided into three stages:

1. In the first, during a hard workout you feel a dull ache in a joint, muscle, tendon, or ligament. The appropriate treatment: Reduce the intensity of your training for one or two days.

2. If hard training is continued, you may feel pain both during and after the workout. At this point, you should rest or try a different sport. If the pain does not improve in a week, seek medical help to determine whether the pain is caused by a structural abnormaility, muscle imbalance, lack of flexibility, or just overwork.

3. Failure to heed the symptoms often will lead to pain even when you are at rest. By this time the only remedy is to stop training entirely until the pain disappears. Often, at this point, you will have to see a physician.

Poor Training Methods

When athletes come to me with injuries, I ask them about their training methods. Rapid increases in workload, speed, and resistance, or adding new training methods to a program often puts more strain on the athletes than their bodies can endure and injures them.

Increasing workload too soon

To train properly, an athlete must stress his body and then allow it to recover. (See Chapter 4.) To improve, you must increase the stress in successive workouts. But to avoid injury, you must increase the stress *gradually*.

A top handball player complained to me about persistent soreness and aching. After examining him, I couldn't find any physical explanation for his problem. "How many times a week do you play?" I asked.

"Until two weeks ago, I was playing four times a week," said the patient. "But now I'm up to six times." His problem: He increased his workload too quickly and his muscles were mildly injured.

Increasing intensity too soon

The heavier the weight you lift or the faster you run, the greater the strain on your body.

A weight lifter came to me with a pulled muscle in his back. In the previous two weeks, he had increased the maximum weight he was pressing in workouts from 260 to 295 pounds. His body couldn't handle the rapid increase in weight. He should have increased his load more gradually — from 260 to 270 to 280 to 295.

A high school runner came to me with a leg injury. He had gone from running his quarter-mile repeats in 72 seconds to running them in 65. He should have increased the speed of his intervals more gradually — from 72 to 70 to 68 to 66 to 65 seconds.

Adding a new training method

Even if you are in top shape, adding a new training method to your program — such as lifting weights or using an isokinetic machine — should be done very gradually. Because of the principle of specificity (see Chapter 4), you will be using your muscles in a different way than you did with your regular workouts.

A football player came to me in August complaining about shin splints. In the week prior to his injury, his coach had instructed him to run up the stadium steps daily. This put added stress on his shin muscles in the front of his leg. His year-round running program had not been not specific enough to develop these muscles and they became injured.

Structural Abnormalities

Structural abnormalities can put extra stress on muscles, fasciae, bones, joints, tendons, or ligaments, and result in injuries to these structures.

Having "flat feet" can cause injuries to the arch, ankle, hip, and lower back.

Having too high an arch can cause stress fractures of the foot and pain on the outside part of your knee.

Having legs of unequal lengths can cause hip and low-back injuries.

Having bowlegs can cause low-back pain.

Having knock-knees can cause pain in the ankle, knee, and hip.

Having an exaggerated curve in your lower back can cause low-back pain.

Excessive Pronation of the Feet

Whenever an athlete comes to me with an injury to his or her legs or back, I examine the feet. I'm looking for a condition that you would call "flat feet." Usually the feet are not flat. They only appear that way because the ankles are weak and allow the feet to roll inward excessively.

To understand why weak ankles cause injuries, you must first understand the normal gait cycle.

When you run, you land first on your heel; as the foot moves forward, your weight transfers to the outside part of your foot. Then your foot rolls inward so that all your weight is shifted to the inside bottom part of your foot. It is this rolling inward, called pronation, that distributes the force of a footstrike throughout the entire foot and leg. Pronation is nature's way of protecting the lower extremities from injury.

Feet that appear to be flat usually roll inward excessively. This is called excessive pronation and it's this condition that is the villain behind many injuries to the ankles, knees, hips, bones, and muscles.

I can easily pick out people who pronate excessively. Their feet appear flat. The outside back of their shoe heels always wears down first, because to compensate for the excessive pronation, these people land too far back on their heels.

The Pronated Foot

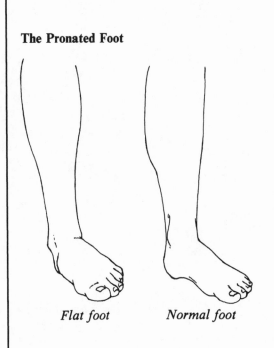

Flat foot   *Normal foot*

The major purpose of athletic shoes is to limit pronation. To accomplish this, a good shoe should have a flared heel for stability and a cookie to support the arch. A stiff Achilles counter, a tight collar, and a good saddle help to stabilize the foot in the shoe. To limit pronation it must fit like a glove. Thick socks prevent the shoe from fitting snugly and should never be worn. I recommend that you wear no socks or thin stretch ones.

Runner's Knee

The most common injury caused by excessive pronation is runner's knee, sometimes also known as basketball knee. According to Joe Henderson, the former editor of *Runner's World*, knee injuries affect 25 percent of all serious runners and most of these injuries are due to runner's knee.

Runner's knee is characterized by pain behind the kneecap during exercise. The excessive pronation exaggerates the normal twisting inward of the lower leg. This, in turn, causes the kneecap to rub painfully against the long bone of the thigh.

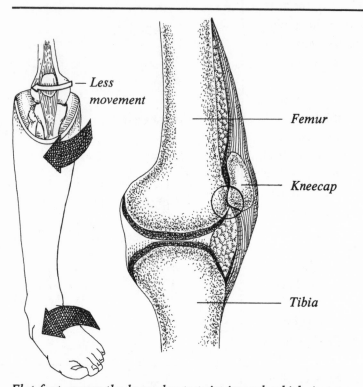

Flat foot causes the lower leg to twist inward, which, in turn, causes the kneecap to rub against the long bone of the thigh.

What to Look For in an Athletic Shoe

Always make sure that the shoe fits your foot. If your foot is a D width, you can probably wear any one of a hundred different running shoes. However, if you have a wide or narrow foot, you must request a shoe that comes in widths.

The sole should be flexible. Bend the shoe. If it does not bend easily, it is too stiff and may cause pain in the bottom of your foot, your Achilles tendon, or your calf muscle.

The shoe should have a cookie to support the arch in your foot. Most running injuries are caused by excessive rolling inward of the foot. A support under your arch limits rolling inward.

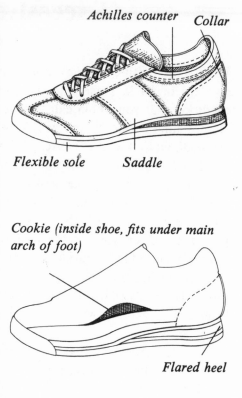

Until 1970, the treatment was to inject cortisone into the knee or to shave the back of the kneecap surgically.

These treatments arose from a basic misconception about the cause of the condition. Runner's knee has been mistakenly termed *Patella Chondromalacia*, which means a softening of the cartilage behind the kneecap.

I've known for years that neither surgery nor cortisone shots help very often. Most of my running friends who have had surgery were never able to compete again.

Orthotics

In 1970, Dr. George Sheehan, a world record holder in the mile for men over fifty (4:47), published a paper in *Runner's World* that revolutionized the treatment of runner's knee and other leg and hip injuries. Dr. Sheehan described the case of Tom Bache, a top cross-country runner, who had runner's knee. His knee failed to respond to two years of standard medical treatment. Finally, John Pagliano, a podiatrist and marathoner, built special inserts called orthotics for Bache's running shoes. The orthotics prevented excessive pronation. Within two weeks Bache was running without pain.

I asked Dr. Sheehan what made him suspect that abnormal foot structure causes knee problems. He said he often had knee pain when he ran on the street with traffic, none when he ran against the traffic. On the with-traffic side, the slope of the road caused his left foot to land higher than his right one. The problem: He was landing on a part of his foot that caused his knee and thigh bones to rub, creating pain. On the other side of the street, the foot position was reversed, and his bones didn't rub together.

An orthotic is a special shoe insert made from a cast of

Orthotics

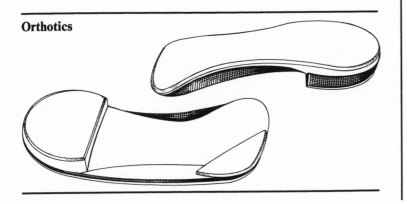

Weight lifter Mark Cameron was afflicted with runner's knee, in his case better labeled weight lifter's knee. His problem came from bad weight lifting form. "Unfortunately I went to a doctor and he put my knee in a cast," says Cameron. "If I knew then what I know now, I never would have gone to a doctor. I would have treated it myself."

Many Athletes Wear Orthotics

Basketball stars Dave Cowens, Doug Collins, and Bob McAdoo all wear orthotics.

Doug Collins, an Olympic basketball star who now plays for the Philadelphia 76ers, "works and plays in his orthotics," according to Dr. Gary Gordon, his podiatrist. He wears them to treat "plantar fasciitis." More than 60 percent of the players on the Los Angeles Lakers and Buffalo Braves wear orthotics.

Skier Pete Patterson uses orthotics. "I really didn't like them that well in the beginning. Now I can't ski without them."

Craig Virgin, National Collegiate Athletic Association cross-country champion, lost two years of running before he obtained his orthotics.

the patient's foot. It looks like an arch support. Acrylic posts under the heel restrict the foot from rolling inward excessively. By preventing the arch from going flat, most painful injuries can be eliminated.

Besides knee problems, orthotics are used to treat certain back, hip, ankle, arch, and foot conditions.

Athletes in many sports now use orthotics. So many players in the National Basketball Association use them that Ray Melchiorre, the trainer for the Buffalo Braves, has heard a player brag, "I faked him out of his orthotics."

Orthotics can be rigid or flexible. Rigid ones offer better foot control, but flexible orthotics usually are preferred by athletes because they are more comfortable and less restrictive.

Orthotics can be obtained from a podiatrist or an orthopedist for $75 to $150. To save money, you may want to try an arch support first. They are not as effective as orthotics in limiting pronation, but they may help. You can buy them for less than $10 at most drugstores.

High-Arched Feet

People with high-arched feet don't pronate enough to distribute the force of the footstrike throughout the entire leg. When a foot pronates normally, the arch falls slightly, causing the knee and the leg to turn inward. It is this motion that absorbs some of the shock of the footstrike. When the arch is rigid, pronation is limited and the entire force of the footstrike is usually transmitted to the bones of the feet and the outside part of the knee and hip. That's why people with high arches develop stress fractures of their feet and pain on the outside part of their knees (lateral knee ligaments) and hips.

The treatment is to cushion the foot with thick-soled shoes fitted with an arch support made from soft, pliable material. People with limited pronation should also run on soft ground and avoid running on hard concrete. Because orthotics will further restrict pronation, they usually are ineffective in treating a high-arched foot.

Bowlegs and Knock-knees

Stand up straight with your heels together. If the space between your knees is greater than the width of two fingers, you are bowlegged and are susceptible to low-back pain.

If you are bowlegged, your iliopsoas muscle, which runs from your pelvis to the upper inner part of your thigh, is usually shortened. When you run, it tilts your pelvis forward. This increases the curvature of your spine and can cause low-back pain. The treatment is to stretch the iliopsoas muscles and to perform all the exercises under back pain in Chapter 10.

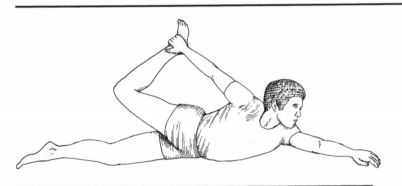

Stand up straight with your knees together. Do you have trouble putting your heels together? If you do, you have knock-knees and are more susceptible to pains on the inner part of your knees. Most people who have this structural abnormality also have excessively pronated feet, which are treated with orthotics. If you are knock-kneed, don't have excessive pronation, and have knee pain, see an orthopedist. In my experience, braces, special shoes, and surgery are often not effective treatments and should be attempted in only the most severe cases. Fortunately, some newly developed surgical techniques may offer benefit to some carefully selected patients.

Unequal Leg Lengths

A difference of as little as ¼ inch between the length of each of your legs can cause pain in the hip, low back, and back of the leg. When one leg is shorter than the other, your pelvis tilts laterally toward the shorter leg, creating pressure and pain on the hip joint of the longer leg. The tilted pelvis also twists the spinal column and shortens the space between the vertebral bodies, which pinches the

Exercise to Stretch the Iliopsoas Muscle

1. Lie on your side.
2. Grab the ankle of your uppermost leg with your hand.
3. Pull the ankle backward and slightly to the side.
4. Hold for the count of ten, then relax.
5. Repeat this stretch ten times.
6. Turn around and repeat exercise with other leg.

Severe side effects of unequal leg lengths

1. An S-shaped curve of the spine
2. One hip higher than the other
3. One shoulder higher than the other

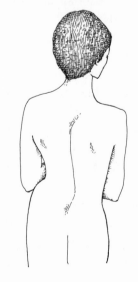

nerves that pass between them. The ligaments that hold the vertebral bodies in place can be strained and cause pain in the back.

To find out if one of your legs is shorter than the other, stand with your heels together. With a tape, measure the distance from the floor to the same spot on each side of the top of the pelvis. If the distances are unequal, so are the lengths of your legs.

The next step is to sit in a chair with your feet on the floor. Put your heels together and point your toes forward. Place a carpenter's level on your knees. If the bubble is not in the middle, the leg length discrepancy is below your knees.

Next, stand up with your heels together and your toes pointed forward. If the small bony protrusions on the inside of your ankle, called *medial malleoli,* are of unequal heights, the discrepancy is below the ankle.

Either you have excessive pronation of one foot or one foot is smaller than the other. If the arch in your shorter leg is flat, you have excessive pronation and you should see an orthopedist or a podiatrist for an orthotic.

If you don't have excessive pronation, ask a cobbler to build up the sole and heel of the shoe you wear on your smaller foot.

Lack of Flexibility

"Stretching is the most important injury preventive in sports today," says Bob Bauman, a trainer for fifty years in professional baseball and college basketball.

Why do Bauman and so many other trainers think so highly of stretching?

They know that when athletes exercise vigorously, their muscles are injured slightly. With healing, the affected muscle becomes shorter and tighter. A tight muscle is more susceptible to injury. That's why athletes who don't stretch lack flexibility and are injured more frequently.

In sports requiring running, the two muscles most commonly victimized by pulls and strains are the hamstrings, in the back of the thigh, and the calf muscles, in the back of the lower leg.

On some professional teams, stretching has reduced these injuries by as much as 80 percent. Athletes, especially those who compete in running sports, should make a regular practice of stretching their muscles.

Most Professional Athletes Stretch

Tennis stars Chris Evert and Arthur Ashe stretch.

Golfer Lee Trevino says that stretching helps to improve his swing and strengthen his back.

Soccer star Kyle Rote, Jr. stretches every day.

Weight lifter Mark Cameron does fifteen minutes of stretching exercises before he even touches a barbell.

Bowler Carmen Salvino stretches his fingers daily so that he can get a better grip on the ball.

The Buffalo Braves have compulsory stretching for twenty minutes a day. "In the last five years we have had only three noncontact muscle strains and the players missed only a few games," says Ray Melchiorre, the trainer.

Many years ago, Carl Yastrzemski, the Boston Red Sox superstar, suffered muscle pulls that forced him to miss a portion of several baseball seasons. Yaz began a stretching program and more than a decade later is still playing great baseball.

Reggie Jackson, the New York Yankees slugger, has the flexibility of a ballet dancer. Despite his huge size, he can perform a split all the way to the ground. His chance of pulling a groin muscle is almost zero.

Football's Pittsburgh Steelers were plagued with muscle pulls and strains a few years ago. After leading the league in injuries, the Steelers hired Paul Uram as a flexibility coach. He evaluated all the players for muscle tightness and, when indicated, recommended stretching exercises. I don't think it was a coincidence that the Steelers were relatively free from injuries and won two Superbowl championships after Uram was added to the coaching staff.

"Four years ago, we eliminated calisthenics and brought in a stretching *(continued)*

If you compete in a sport that requires running, I recommend that you perform the four stretching exercises on p. 140 before each workout or competition and before you go to bed. Repeat each exercise at least five times.

What about the athlete who is so tight that a stretching program is not successful?

Dr. James Nicholas, team physician for the New York Jets, tells a story about Jim Wise, who now plays for the Minnesota Vikings. "His inner thigh muscles were so tight that he repeatedly pulled his groin muscles even though he tried a stretching program. I had to put him in traction in the hospital so his legs would be constantly stretched. In three days, I was able to stretch his legs ten inches further apart. He stopped having groin pulls."

coach from San Diego," declares Tim Davey of the New York Jets. "Since then there has been a magnificent decrease in injuries."

Nowadays, most National Football League teams hire a flexibility coach who evaluates the players and assigns corrective exercises to those with tight muscles.

Muscle Imbalance

Lee Burkitt of Arizona State University can predict athletic injuries before they happen. He has done it for the San Diego Charger professional football team and for competitive trackmen. Is Burkitt a mystic? Hardly. He's a scientist who has studied muscle imbalance.

When a muscle moves in one direction, another muscle moves in the opposite direction. These muscles are called opposing muscles. The ratio of strength between opposing muscles is delicately balanced. If one of the muscles is much stronger than the other, an imbalance exists. The stronger muscle can overpower the weaker one, causing damage to its fibers and tendons. The treatment for muscle imbalance is to strengthen the weaker muscle and to stretch the stronger one.

Pulled hamstrings

A hamstring pull is a common athletic injury and is usually due to muscle imbalance. The hamstring muscle, located in the back of the thigh, lowers the knee. Its opposing muscle is the quad, a massive muscle in the front of the thigh which raises the knee.

Burkitt, using a gauge to measure muscle strength, discovered that most athletes in sports requiring running have quads that are 1½ times stronger than their hamstrings. Those athletes who had a higher strength ratio between these two muscles were the ones most likely to pull their hamstrings.

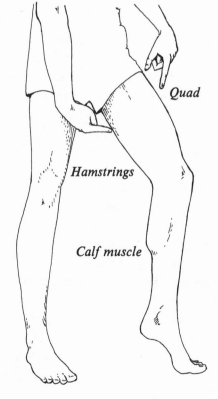

Quad

Hamstrings

Calf muscle

Four Important Stretching Exercises

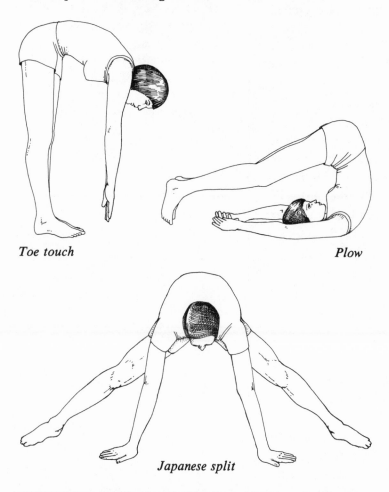

Toe touch

Plow

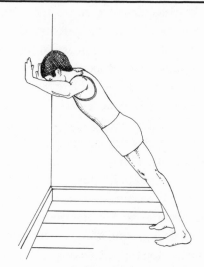

Wall push-up

Japanese split

Athletes who have a lower ratio almost never pull their hamstrings. Skiers, skaters, and cyclists are good examples; because they never fully straighten their knees, their hamstrings are almost as strong as their quads. Runners, bowlers, and football, soccer, and basketball players, because they always straighten their knees, often have greater strength ratios and frequently injure their hamstrings.

Why does straightening your knee make you more susceptible to hamstring injuries?

David Kelley, a professor of kinesiology (the study of how muscles work) at the University of Maryland, gave me the following explanation: "The hamstrings are two-joint muscles. When they contract, they both straighten the hip joint and bend the knee joint. When the hip joint is bent and the knee joint is straightened, as occurs during the running cycle, great tension is exerted on the hamstrings. So much so that fibers can be torn. At this point the great tension also stretches the muscle with such force that the

Wall push-up to stretch the calves: Face a wall, standing at least four feet away. Place your palms on the wall, keeping your back straight. Bend your elbows so your upper body will move closer to the wall. If you keep your heels on the ground, the calves and Achilles tendons will be stretched. Hold this position to the count of ten. Straighten your elbows. Then repeat at least five times.

Toe-touching to stretch the hamstrings: With your heels together and knees straight, try to touch the ground or floor with your fingers. Do not bounce. Hold the position to the count of ten. Release, then repeat at least five times.

The plow to stretch the lower back and hamstrings: Lie on your back. Without bending your knees, raise your legs over your head and try to touch the ground with your toes. Do not force. Hold to the count of ten. Lower your legs and repeat at least five times.

Japanese split to stretch the inner thighs: Stand erect. Without bending your knees, gradually spread your legs apart as far as you can. Place your palms on the floor for balance. Hold your maximum stretch for at least ten seconds. Repeat at least five times.

hamstrings do not contract like a muscle. Instead, they are stretched like a tendon."

Logically, you would think that the treatment for hamstring injuries would be to stretch the stronger muscle (the quad) and to strengthen the weaker one (the hamstrings). However, the treatment for hamstring injuries is unique because the hamstrings function as both a muscle and a tendon. Since the treatment for a muscle injury is strengthening and for a tendon injury is stretching, the treatment for a hamstring pull is both strengthening and stretching it. The hamstring has an upper part that straightens the hip and a lower part that bends the knee, and both parts must be strengthened. You should not start your corrective program until the muscle has healed. This usually takes a week or longer.

To stretch your hamstrings, perform the plow and toe-touching exercises described earlier in this chapter.

Hamstring Pulls Should Be Prevented

Because Paul Uram, the Steeler's flexibility coach, understands muscle imbalance, he uses corrective exercises and in five years has had only one player miss a game due to a hamstring pull.

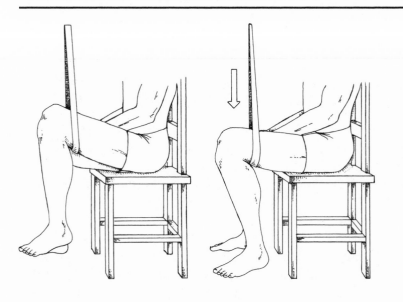

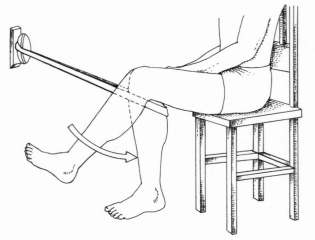

To Strengthen the Upper Hamstrings

1. Bolt an innertube firmly to a post or a door molding so that the bottom of the tube is 6 inches above the top of your knee when you are seated in a straight chair.
2. Put the leg closest to the tube through it so that the bottom rests under your thigh.
3. Forcefully lower your foot to the ground, then relax. Repeat rapidly ten times. Rest 30 seconds. Repeat procedure five times.
4. Repeat with other leg.

To Strengthen the Lower Hamstrings

1. Fasten one end of a bicycle innertube to a stationary object such as a doorknob.
2. Sit down and put one leg through the other end, as pictured in the diagram. The innertube should be tightly stretched.
3. Bend the knee backward rapidly ten times, increasing tension on the tube. Rest for 30 seconds. Repeat the procedure five times.
4. Repeat with the other leg.

Shin splints

Shin splints are another condition that can result from muscle imbalance. They are characterized by generalized pain in front of the lower leg and are particularly common in runners and running backs. Shin splints are due to injured muscles, and should be differentiated from a crack in the bone, or a pinched-off blood supply. To do this takes special medical knowledge. For this reason, shin splints that don't respond within three weeks to the treatment recommended here should be checked by a physician. The most common cause is a muscle imbalance where the calf muscles — which pull the forefoot down — overpower the shin muscles — which pull the forefoot up. As the athlete continues to train, the calf muscle usually becomes proportionately much stronger than the shin muscles.

The treatment for shin splints is to strengthen the weaker muscles (shins) and stretch the stronger muscles (calves).

To strengthen the shins, run up stairs. To stretch the calves, either use the inclined plane described in Chapter 9 or wall push-ups, described earlier in this chapter.

Warming Up

Always warm up before you exercise. Warming up increases the blood supply to the muscles and raises their temperature. This, in turn, makes them more pliable and resistant to injury.

Don't waste your time with calisthenics. Almost all the professional teams we interviewed have stopped doing them. They don't stretch your tight muscles, don't strengthen your weak ones, and don't even use your muscles in the same manner you will use them when you exercise.

I recommend that your warm-up be done in two phases. First, stretch the muscles that are tight from previous exercise. If your sport requires running, perform the stretching exercises on page 140. If you are a weight lifter, do the stretches for runners and also stretch your arms, shoulders, and back.

Next, warm up your muscles by exercising them in the same way as when you participate in your sport. Start off slowly and gradually increase the intensity of your exercise. Hockey players should skate around the rink ten to

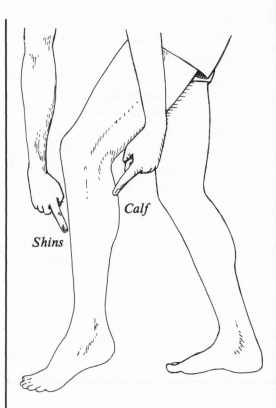

Calf

Shins

Spencer Haywood of the New York Knicks had a nagging case of shin splints that didn't respond to a stretching program. He went to Dr. Don O'Donoghue, who diagnosed it as a blocked blood supply and operated. Haywood is now able to play basketball again.

Robin Campbell, one of the top female runners in the United States, suffered from shin splints a few months before the 1976 Olympics and lost her chance for a medal.

"I knew that the only cure for shin splints was rest, but the Olympic trials come up only once every four years," says Miss Campbell. "It hurt to run, but I competed and made it to the semi-finals."

Like pulled hamstrings, shin splints need time to heal. Doctors treated Robin with stretching and strengthening exercises, but until she rested, the shin splints wouldn't heal.

fifteen times before a game. Runners should jog slowly for the first few minutes. Tennis players should rally for ten minutes. The key to a good warm-up is to increase the pace of your workout so gradually that your muscles can adjust to the increased pace and remain free from injury.

12.

Exercising in Extreme Weather

Ten Fallacies about Hot Weather

Even on the hottest day of the year, I run. Competing or exercising in the heat is dangerous only if you don't understand or don't follow the basic principles of hot-weather exercise. To help protect you from mistakes that are commonly made by athletes and fitness buffs, I have prepared a list of ten common fallacies. By avoiding these fallacies, you can participate safely and compete more effectively in your sport when the heat is on.

Fallacy 1. You don't need extra conditioning to exercise in the heat

Nothing can be further from the truth. It takes a higher level of conditioning to exercise in the heat. I know many runners who can compete effectively in the winter on a training program of only thirty-five miles a week. But in the hot weather, that amount of training is not adequate.

During exercise every muscle is a tiny furnace that produces heat. In cold weather, that heat is carried by the bloodstream to the skin where it is dissipated in the cool air through four means: radiation, evaporation, convection, and conduction. However, in the summer when the temperature difference between the skin and the air is small, only evaporation can effectively dissipate body heat. This evaporation takes place through sweating.

"The Holyoke Massacre"

It was called the Holyoke Massacre by runners who competed in the 1967 marathon in 97-degree heat. Many of the kings of distance running had assembled in Holyoke, Massachusetts, to determine, in a 26-mile national A.A.U. championship race, who would represent the United States that year in the Pan American Games. One by one, "sun power" beat most of them down. At the end, 87 of 125 well-conditioned runners were unable to finish.

Ron Daws, a runner who was not expected to be among the leaders, finished first. He describes his extraordinary upset win:

"At nineteen miles, I spotted Tom Laris, the pre-race favorite, weaving along at the side of the road. I quickened my pace to overtake him. I never got the honor. Tom quit before I could pass him, claiming afterwards that his health was more important. I won not because I was inherently the better runner, but because on that day I was able to cope with the heat."

Daws learned how to prepare for
(continued)

The higher the humidity and temperature, the more slowly sweat evaporates.

Your body has three million sweat glands — tubes that draw fluid from the blood to produce sweat and then transport it through the pores to the skin surface. To compensate for the lower efficiency of evaporation in hot weather, your body sweats over a greater percentage of your skin surface. That's the reason that in the summer you sweat over your entire body surface and in the winter you sweat primarily from your face and chest.

In hot weather, your heart must work harder to supply more blood to a greater surface area of skin. Thus, a higher level of fitness is required.

Fallacy 2. You don't need to train specifically to exercise in heat and high humidity

To compete effectively in the heat, you must sweat heavily in training. Acclimatization — getting your body accustomed to hot weather — takes up to two weeks. The watchwords: Get ready, get set, sweat!

Acclimatization teaches your body to sweat better. It enlarges the sweat glands so that they can produce more sweat and widens the blood vessels in the skin so more blood can be carried to the surface of the skin and its heat can be dissipated by evaporation.

When you exercise under the hot sun with your shirt off, you may not sweat heavily enough to enlarge your sweat glands and widen your blood vessels. You will not acclimatize as well as someone training in cold weather with many sweat suits.

Fallacy 3. You can perform as well in the heat as in the cold

Hot weather saps a competitor's strength, cuts endurance, and plays havoc with performance.

In hot weather, any endurance athlete should expect his performance to be below par. A marathoner, for example, should add five to fifteen minutes to his expected time and pace himself accordingly. Butch Buchholz claims a tennis player who can boom a serve in at a hundred miles per hour may lose up to fifteen miles per hour in the heat.

Every athlete, when competing in the heat, sooner or later learns to hold back early so he'll have something left

hot-weather competition the hard way. Three years earlier in the Yonkers Marathon, which determined the members of the 1964 U.S. Olympic team, the race began at high noon in 96-degree heat.

"At the twenty-fifth mile, cramps so paralyzed my legs that I lurched for the telephone pole and embraced it for support," recalls Daws. "I had to be hospitalized."

After recovering, Daws was determined to find out how Buddy Edelen had won the race by more than twenty minutes, one of the widest margins ever in a major marathon. How could he run so well in hot weather when he lived and trained in England with 50-degree temperatures during the two months preceding the Olympic trials?

Edelen's secret: He trained in five layers of clothing which made him sweat heavily. The increased sweating taught his body how to handle the heat.

Daws immediately picked up on Edelen's technique and thereafter trained heavily clothed.

On the day of the Holyoke Marathon, Daws recalls, "I smiled to myself when I saw Tom Laris sporting a beautiful tan. He had been training in nothing more than his shoes and his shorts."

"Being Hit with a Stick"

"Exercising under the hot sun is like being hit with a stick," says marathoner Tom Osler, a top hot-weather performer. "You will never become accustomed to being beaten with a stick. So it is with those who train under the hot sun."

in reserve. The heat of summer is no time to set records. Here are the reasons:

> Your heart must work harder. In addition to pumping blood to your muscles, your heart must increase the amount of blood it pumps to the skin.
>
> Your muscles do not work as efficiently. Exercise in hot weather impairs performance by increasing fluid loss and raising your body and muscle temperature. When their temperature rises, muscles don't extract oxygen, produce energy, or contract efficiently.
>
> It takes more calories to exercise in the heat. The extra workload on your heart requires more energy. Your heart burns more calories than any other muscle in your body. Since it must work harder in hot weather, your caloric requirements increase.

Fallacy 4. You can replace salt lost in sweat by taking salt tablets

Never — I repeat, never — take salt tablets. You get more than enough salt from the salt shaker, meats, and other foods. In fact, federal government researchers say the average American diet contains too much salt.

When sweating, you lose proportionately more water than salt, leaving a higher level of sodium or salt in the bloodstream. Popping salt tablets simply elevates the level further and, in the opinion of many medical authorities, increases the chances of heatstroke.

Heavy concentrations of salt thicken your blood and make it more likely to clot. Clots can cause a heart attack, stroke, kidney failure, blindness, and even death. For a healthy person, taking too much salt is more dangerous than not taking enough.

If your body requires extra salt, you will crave it. Consequently, you will prefer salty foods and will use the salt shaker more.

Of all the minerals, salt is the least understood by athletes. For a more complete discussion, see Chapter 7.

Fallacy 5. Salt (sodium) is the only mineral you need in hot weather

This is ridiculous. An acclimatized athlete loses almost no salt in his sweat and urine in hot weather. Potassium, not salt, is the mineral that the body needs most.

After you stop exercising, you must replace your potassium by eating fruits and vegetables and drinking fruit

"Picking Them Off Like Flies"

In the 1967 Holyoke Massacre, forty-two-year-old Jim McDonough felt that patience was his best bet in competing against so many star performers for one of the top spots that would qualify him to represent this country in the Pan American Games.

So he started out very slowly. By holding a steady pace, he passed every runner in the race, except one. It wasn't that he was accelerating. The other runners slowed down so much that he picked them off like flies.

The fast early pace of other runners had destroyed them. McDonough's patience in the heat earned him a second-place finish and a place on the U.S. team.

Frank Challant, the Boston Celtics trainer, told me that one rookie took so many salt tablets that he became sick. He vomited, developed stomach cramps, and became extremely weak. Because the extra salt deprived the player's body of potassium and fluid, Challant treated him with bananas and a gallon of water.

Filling Up on Potassium

"You don't usually have to worry about potassium unless athletes aren't eating their fruits," says swimming coach Doc Counsilman.

"I try to eat lots of fruits for its potassium content," says weight lifter Mark Cameron.

"I eat bananas for potassium," relates Kyle Rote, Jr.

"The more I wrestle, the more fruit I eat," says Olympic champion Dan Gable.

juices. If you don't you will soon become exhausted and suffer "the mineral blues." (See Chapter 7.)

During exercise each muscle produces heat. To control heat buildup, the muscle releases potassium into its veins. Potassium causes the veins to widen and increases the circulation of blood through the muscle. The increased circulation carries away more heat and cools the muscle. Thus, during exercise in hot weather, the bloodstream contains increased amounts of potassium.

Because increased amounts of potassium in the blood can interfere with the ability of your heart to contract, the body quickly eliminates it through your urine and sweat. During hard exercise, your body can excrete ten times as much potassium in the sweat and urine as during rest. This lost potassium must be replaced.

Fallacy 6. Never swallow liquids during competition; just rinse out your mouth

On the contrary, you should drink as much as you can.

The body loses tremendous amounts of fluid during heavy exercise and competition, particularly in hot weather. You not only sweat, but with every breath you emit water vapor from your lungs.

On a hot day, a bicycle racer or a soccer player can lose ten pounds of fluid. A basketball player can lose from five to ten pounds, and a marathoner can lose up to fourteen pounds. Most of this weight loss is due to sweat.

The intelligent athlete drinks all the time. But no matter how much he drinks, he won't be able to keep pace with his fluid losses during competition. In heavy continuous hot-weather exercise, an athlete can sweat and breathe away four pounds of water an hour.

If you engage in intense exercise on a hot day, drink a cup or two of liquid fifteen to twenty minutes after you start to exercise and continue to drink the same amount every fifteen minutes. If you take more than two cups at one time, the fluid may distend your stomach, which may press on your diaphragm and make breathing uncomfortable.

You shouldn't wait for thirst before you drink because your body loses two to four pounds of fluid before you feel thirsty. Here's why: When you sweat you lose proportionately more water than salt, leaving a higher level of salt in the bloodstream. It is this increased concentration of salt in your blood that signals the osmoreceptors, small cells in your brain, to tell you that you are thirsty. You must lose a

In the Heat, Athletes Lose Tremendous Amounts of Fluid

On a hot day, Philadelphia pitcher Larry Christenson and soccer star Kyle Rote, Jr. can lose twelve pounds; tennis player Butch Buchholz, ten pounds; and basketball stars Calvin Murphy, five pounds, and Paul Silas, seventeen pounds. In the 1968 Olympic marathon trials, Ron Daws lost nine pounds, or 6 percent of his body weight, despite drinking fluids every two miles. Most of this weight loss is due to sweat.

In Hot Weather, Drink, Drink, Drink

Most coaches and trainers encourage their athletes to drink at every time-out or break in the action. In sports like boxing, baseball, and football, athletes can drink between rounds, in the dugout, or on the sidelines. Cyclists take fluids from their squeeze bottles every fifteen minutes. Marathon runners try to drink at every station, 2½ miles apart. Even skier Tim Caldwell, who competes in cold weather, drinks liquids every fifteen to twenty minutes during a race.

"Everytime we pass our own bench, we sneak ice cubes," relates Bobby Moffat of the Dallas Tornado.

large amount of fluid before the salt concentration in your bloodstream rises enough to affect the osmoreceptors.

If you compete in sports requiring continuous movement, such as running, cycling, and cross-country skiing, you should drink a glass of water ten minutes before competition. If you drink more than ten minutes before competition, the water will pass through your kidneys and fill your bladder. It's uncomfortable to exercise with a full bladder. However, once you start to exercise, your body stops producing urine. Your muscles require so much blood that the heart sends most of the blood to your muscles and skin and very little to your kidneys.

Fallacy 7. During competition or exercise, commercially prepared drinks are best

Not true. Most commercial drinks sold in stores, both the carbonated kind and those that are advertised as mineral-replacement drinks for athletes, contain too much sugar to be used during competition. Scientists have determined that the ideal drink should contain less than 2.5 percent sugar. Drinks containing greater concentrations than that are absorbed poorly by the intestinal tract and tend to remain in the stomach for longer periods of time. They can cause bloating, cramping, and discomfort. The main purpose of putting sugar into athletic drinks is to make them taste good.

For sports requiring intense continuous muscular exercise, the sugar in drinks doesn't help much anyway. Much more sugar is being burned by the muscles than could possibly be replaced by a sugared drink. Therefore, these drinks should be considered only as a source of fluid, not a source of sugar. Thus a marathon runner, soccer player, or basketball player should use these drinks only if they have been diluted one part of the commercial drink with two or three parts water. Orange juice, an excellent athletic drink, should be diluted in the same proportion.

Athletes in sports that do not require intense or continuous exercise can drink heavily sugared drinks without cramping or discomfort. Baseball games, for example, can last several hours. Because the players are not running continuously, large amounts of sugared drinks will not cause stomach cramps. The reason: The muscles don't compete with the stomach for the blood supply. Gene Monahan of the New York Yankees makes up a "Monahan special" of orange juice and honey that team members drink between innings.

Too Much Sugar

In the 1968 Olympic marathon trials, Billy Mills, the defending Olympic champion at 10,000 meters, developed severe muscle cramps after drinking a large quantity of a heavily sugared commercial drink, and failed to make the team.

Drinks after competition are another story. They should be loaded with minerals and carbohydrates. That's when the body needs them most. The most popular drink for every sport we checked was beer — high in minerals and calories.

I recommend orange or other fruit juices. Not only do they contain much-needed potassium, they also have trace minerals that are also necessary for normal body functions.

Fallacy 8. Drink tepid liquids because they are absorbed into the bloodstream more quickly

Strange as it may seem, cold drinks increase motility and are absorbed faster than warm drinks. In recent years, Cyril Wyndham, a physician in South Africa, has shown that drinks are absorbed best at a temperature of 40°.

I was mistakenly told in medical school that consuming cold drinks during exercise causes cramps. I once tried to drink warm water during a race, but it tasted so bad that I never again drank warm beverages during competition.

Every professional team ices down drinks during competition. Not one athlete that we interviewed ever had stomach cramps from cold drinks. In fact, a large number of soccer and hockey players told us they regularly chew ice.

Fallacy 9. During competition wear as little clothing as possible so air can get to your skin and increase evaporation

This is a half truth. If you're competing under the bright sun, you must wear enough clothing to protect you from its rays. The reason: By heating and even burning your skin, the sun's rays can make you tired. On the other hand, if you wear too much clothing, evaporation is restricted.

The best clothing should be solid enough to block the sun's rays and porous enough to allow evaporation. That's why many athletes wear the porous nylon mesh shirts that can be bought in most sporting goods stores.

Wear white clothing to reflect the sun's rays. Dark clothing absorbs heat.

Covering your head is a must. Have you ever seen a baseball player go on to the field without a cap? It protects his head from the direct rays of the sun.

Knowledgeable marathon runners and cyclists wear hats and pour water on them. As the water evaporates from the

Temperatures as high as 135° have been recorded in the cabs of racing cars. To combat these severe temperatures, some NASCAR drivers wear a Freon-cooled skullcap under their crash helmets. But Buddy Baker says these cooling devices have a drawback. "It cools the head all right, but the rest of the body is hot. It's this temperature imbalance that gives me chills."

hat, it cools the head, where 20 percent of your body heat is lost.

Fallacy 10. Take amphetamines: They get you "up" for top performance

Nothing could be further from the truth. Coupled with hot weather, amphetamines can be lethal. Numerous athletes in many sports have died from hot-weather pill-popping.

Tom Simpson, the best professional cyclist in England in the mid-1960s, once said in defense of amphetamines, "When you get up in the morning, do you need a cup of coffee to get started? After pedaling 150 miles the day before, we might need three or four coffees."

A year later, in the 1967 Tour de France race held in 90-degree heat, Simpson's "coffee" caught up with him. He felt bad at the start, telling friends he had been too "nervous" to sleep. During the thirteenth lap — a 6,000-foot climb up a brutal hill — Simpson began zigzagging across the road far short of the summit and finally collapsed into a coma. He was pronounced dead on arrival at a nearby hospital.

An autopsy showed that he was heavily drugged with amphetamines. A vial of the drug was found in his pocket at the time of his death, according to Bill Gilbert's report in *Sports Illustrated.*

A Danish cyclist who took amphetamines died in the 1960 Olympics. Because the drug made him impervious to pain, the cyclist ignored the early signs of heatstroke — hot pokerlike burning in the chest and muscle, extreme shortness of breath, light-headedness, and blurred vision — and rode on to his death.

Hot-Weather Perils

There's a room in my office with almost a hundred trophies won in races since 1965.

One trophy, however, is far more dear to me than all the rest. It was my first and it says: "Four Mile Run 1965." It could have been my tombstone, because I almost died in that race.

In 1964, while completing a medical fellowship at Johns Hopkins, I decided to become a distance runner at age twenty-nine, after a ten-year layoff.

By June, I had been training and racing for nine months, but had never won a trophy.

As I waited at the starting line for the race in Arlington, Virginia, the midafternoon sun pushed the temperature to over 90 degrees. I noticed many of the top runners were absent and I should have suspected that something was amiss. It was my first race in the heat and at that time I knew nothing about competing in hot weather.

The transition from my air-conditioned home to the hot sun made me uncomfortable. Relying on medical texts, I had taken salt tablets daily. Since I had a chance to win my first trophy, I decided an "upper" would help and I took a 10-milligram amphetamine tablet an hour before the race. (That was my first and last amphetamine.)

As I checked out the competition, I noticed that I was the only runner without a white hat or handkerchief on my head. Foolishly, I had felt the extra weight would slow me down.

Right from the sound of the starter's gun, I pushed the pace. Several runners who had beaten me earlier were taking it easy. I thought they just couldn't keep up.

Early in the race, I passed Hugh Jascourt of Greenbelt, Maryland, the race director. I heard someone mumble to him about no water on the course. At three miles, I forced myself up to seventh place. Trophies were to be given to the top five.

I was not feeling well. My muscles were afire

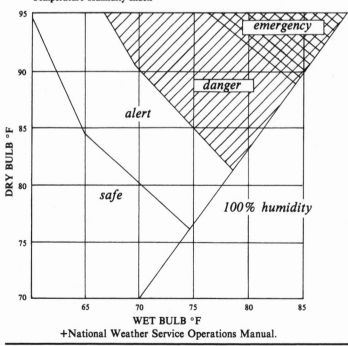

Temperature-Humidity Index

DRY BULB °F

95
90
85
80
75
70

WET BULB °F

65   70   75   80   85

emergency

danger

alert

safe

100% humidity

+National Weather Service Operations Manual.

When Is It Too Hot to Exercise?

Three factors determine the severity of a hot day: temperature, humidity, and wind speed.

When the outside temperature soars to 90° F. or more and the humidity climbs close to 90 percent with little or no wind velocity, there's the ever-present danger of heatstroke and heat exhaustion. Even though it doesn't measure wind speed, the simplest method of measuring the danger of hot day is with a combination wet and dry bulb thermometer. One thermometer, a standard one, measures air temperature; the other, covered by a wick that is dipped in water, is used to measure humidity. They can be bought at any hardware store and usually cost less than $10.00.

By using the Temperature-Humidity Index graph at left, you can determine how dangerous it will be to exercise in the heat.

Read the wet bulb thermometer and record the point on the horizontal axis of the accompanying graph. Record the reading of the dry bulb thermometer on the vertical axis.

and my breath was labored from a burning feeling in my chest. My head started to ache and my feet were full of blisters. My mouth was parched and my tongue seemed to block my breathing.

We came up over a hill and I saw the finish line five hundred yards away. If I could catch two runners seventy yards ahead of me, I would have my trophy.

George Cushmac of Arlington, Virginia, was just ahead of me. I had never beaten him and was surprised to be so close. Drawing on my meager reserve, I broke into a sprint. George looked at me strangely as I went by. He didn't even try to hold me off.

My head was throbbing and I began seeing spots, but I pushed on.

As I neared Bruce Robinson I could hear him moaning and gasping. I stifled my wheezing so he wouldn't know how I was suffering and eased past him into fifth place.

As I hit the finish line, I lost my vision and fell to the ground. I knew something was seriously wrong. I couldn't breathe. My muscles burned. I had the most painful headache of my life.

My temperature must have been 110 degrees. I called for people to pour water on me. But no water was available. I lost consciousness, a victim of heatstroke.

With life-saving presence of mind, my wife had me carried to the shade and put me in shock position — feet elevated, head down. She poured our baby's milk over me. Others doused me with soft drinks and beer. Ice and water were obtained finally from a house nearby and the ice was rubbed on my skin.

After what my wife called an eternity, I awoke. My muscles were so tight I couldn't walk. To receive my fifth-place trophy, I had to be carried to the stand. It was a full three weeks before I could run again.

I know how lucky I am. A few years earlier, two high school runners had died of heatstroke during a ten-mile race in Virginia. Five years earlier, a cyclist died of heatstroke in the Olympics. Each August, football players die of heatstroke during practice.

Heatstroke

Heatstroke is the sudden uncontrolled rise in body temperature caused by the inability of the temperature-regulating

The American College of Sports Medicine Position Statement on the Prevention of Heat Injuries During Distance Running

1. Distance Races (> 16 km. or 10 miles) should *not* be conducted when the wet bulb temperature-wind temperature* exceeds 28° C. (82.4° F.).

2. During the periods of the year when the daylight dry bulb temperature often exeeds 27° C. (80° F.), distance races should be conducted before 9:00 A.M. or after 4:00 P.M.

3. It is the responsibility of the race sponsors to provide fluids which contain small amounts of sugar (less than 2.5 g glucose per 100 cc. of water) and electrolytes (less than 10 mEq sodium and 5 mEq potassium per liter of solution).

4. Runners should be encouraged to ingest fluids frequently during competition and to consume 2 glasses of fluid 10-15 minutes before competition.

5. Rules prohibiting the administration of fluids during the first 10 kilometers (6.2 miles) of a marathon race should be amended to permit fluid ingestion at frequent intervals along the race course. In light of the high sweat rates and body temperatures during distance running in the heat, race sponsors should provide "water stations" at 3-4 kilometer (2-2.5 mile) intervals for all races of 16 kilometers (10 miles) or more.

6. Runners should be instructed in how to recognize the early warning symptoms that precede heat injury. Recognition of symptoms, cessation of running, and proper treatment

*Adapted from Minard, D. Prevention of heat casualties in Marine Corps Recruits. Milit. Med. 126:261, 1961. WB - GT = 0.7 (WBT) + 0.2 (GT) + 0.1 (DBT)

(continued)

cells in the brain to increase the body's mechanisms of dissipating heat.

Normally these brain cells maintain your body temperature close to 98.6° F. They respond primarily to the temperature of the blood that passes through them, and when the temperature of the blood rises, they send signals through nerves to all parts of the body. This widens blood vessels near the surface of the skin so that more heat is given off, and decreases metabolic processes in internal organs so that less heat is produced.

Yet there is a point where the brain cells become damaged by the heat and lose their ability to function. The result: a heatstroke.

The greater your degree of dehydration, the more likely you are to develop heatstroke. The harder you exercise, the less dehydration you can tolerate. Dehydration decreases blood volume to the point where there's not enough blood to supply both the skin and internal organs such as the brain, liver, and muscles. Your body must make a choice and chooses the internal organs and muscles. Thus, the blood supply to the skin is shut off and your body temperature rises uncontrollably.

Heatstroke doesn't just happen. There's plenty of warning. Your lungs and muscles "catch fire." Your breathing becomes short and labored, and your mouth becomes parched. Your vision blurs, and dizziness and nausea set in. You may even start to think and act irrationally. One runner tried to punch me when I was trying to cool him.

If you continue to exercise, you stop sweating and your skin will become dry. It feels dry and clammy even though your body temperature may shoot up to 110° F. You will then become unconscious and unless you receive treatment immediately, you may die for these reasons:

At this point your brain is being cooked and can be destroyed.

Your blood volume, which is already less than normal, continues to decrease. You can lose so much fluid that there is not enough in your bloodstream to support circulation and you go into shock.

The elevated temperature in your blood keeps it from clotting and blood leaks from the blood vessels into your brain, liver, kidneys, and heart and can damage them.

If you suspect that a person is suffering from heatstroke, call for medical help immediately. The victim can die before help arrives. Because the body's temperature is rising rapidly, you don't have much time.

can prevent heat injury. Early warning symptoms include the following: piloerection on chest and upper arms, chilling, throbbing pressure in head, unsteadiness, nausea, and dry skin.

7. Race sponsors should make prior arrangements with medical personnel for the care of cases of heat injury. Responsible and informed personnel should supervise each "feeding station." Organizational personnel should reserve the right to stop runners who exhibit clear signs of heatstroke or heat exhaustion.

It is the position of the American College of Sports Medicine that policies established by local, national, and international sponsors of distance running events should adhere to these guidelines. Failure to adhere to these guidelines may jeopardize the health of competitors through heat injury.

SOURCE: *Medicine and Science in Sports,* volume 7, no. 1, pp. vii–ix, 1975. Copyright 1975, the American College of Sports Medicine. Reprinted by permission.

Place the victim in the shock position with his head down and his legs elevated. The shock position will guarantee a supply of blood to the brain. Pour a lot of liquid — any liquid — all over the victim's body. Promoting evaporation is the key to lowering body temperature. Rubbing ice cubes on the skin is even more effective. Rubbing opens up the blood vessels in the skin and ice is more cooling than water.

Stop the treatment when the victim is wide awake, alert, and out of pain. If you continue the treatment after he is alert, you may drop his body temperature sharply and kill him.

Continue to watch the victim for at least an hour. If he becomes unconscious again, or starts to complain of headache, nausea, or dizziness, repeat the treatment. Several times I have revived patients and while they were talking to me, they have suddenly gone into convulsions, acted irrationally, or lapsed back into unconsciousness. This signals that their temperature is rising again. You must restart treatment and may have to repeat this procedure several times.

If a heatstroke victim doesn't revive in minutes, he may be dying. At this point, a trained medical person must administer special fluids into his veins. After the victim has been revived, he should be encouraged to drink large amounts of fruit juices and other potassium-rich drinks to replace fluids and minerals.

Heatstroke usually occurs in the early spring when athletes and fitness enthusiasts have not had time to acclimatize to the heat. It occurs most frequently on days when both the temperature and the relative humidity are high. High humidity slows the evaporation of sweat.

A victim of heatstroke is more likely to develop another one if he or she exercises vigorously again within a month. After that period, he or she is no more susceptible than others.

Heat Exhaustion

Heat exhaustion is due to loss of water. Unlike heatstroke, which strikes suddenly, heat exhaustion usually comes on over several days. The early symptoms are tiredness, weakness, and malaise. As your body dehydrates, you become progressively weaker until you don't even have the strength to get out of bed. If you continue to lose fluid, your blood volume decreases to the point where you may go into shock.

This is how it happens. Sixty-five percent of your body weight is fluid, which is stored in three compartments: 56 percent inside your cells, 37 percent outside your cells, and 7 percent in your bloodstream. When you first lose water by sweating, breathing, and urinating, almost all of it is lost from inside your cells. Thus, even though you may be lacking as much as eight glasses of water, your cells can supply enough water so that your blood volume remains normal.

If you continue to lose water, your cells reach a point where they are unable to give up any more water and your blood volume drops. When this happens, you may not have enough blood volume to circulate effectively through your body, your temperature rises, and you can go into shock. Fortunately, this catastrophe rarely happens unless you are unable to obtain any fluid replacement.

Usually heat exhaustion is not an emergency condition, but when you exercise you will be more susceptible to heatstroke.

The treatment for heat exhaustion is to drink large amounts of mineral-rich fluid such as fruit juice.

Why do so many athletes lose tremendous amounts of fluid during exercise and rarely suffer heat exhaustion?

For one reason, their bodies can operate on lower levels of fluid. Their hearts pump blood more efficiently and their blood vessels direct the blood flow more efficiently to vital areas.

Secondly, experienced athletes and fitness enthusiasts are very aware of their need to replace fluid all the time, before, during, and after exercise.

Heat exhaustion with too much salt

If an athlete takes salt tablets when his body has too little salt, it will help retain water. However, if he takes salt tablets when his body has normal amounts or too much salt, it will cause him to lose an increased amount of water as well as potassium.

An overdose of salt can be more harmful than a lack of it.

Having too much salt in your blood is the most critical form of heat exhaustion, because it is the one most likely to kill.

Excess salt thickens the blood, making it more likely to clot. A blood clot raises havoc in the body: in the kidney it

Too Much Salt

In the 1978 Superstars competition, Guy Druit, the 1976 Olympic gold medalist in the 110-meter hurdles, and Franz Klammer, the Olympic champion in downhill skiing, both suffered from heat exhaustion. Each collapsed in competition after he had downed a dozen salt tablets.

Tommy Woodcock, the trainer, treated Druit and Klammer with large amounts of a drink full of potassium. He also put them in a cool room and elevated their feet.

can lead to kidney failure; in the heart it can lead to a heart attack; in the brain it can cause a stroke.

Normally, your taste buds protect you from getting too much salt. When there's too much salt in your system, salty foods taste repulsive. But salt tablets bypass the taste-bud mechanism and you don't know when to stop taking them.

Kevin A., a sixteen-year-old football player, had heat exhaustion from taking too much salt. The details of his case should help others avoid making the same mistakes.

In August he started his own training routine — calisthenics and running twice a day. Because he sweated copiously, he took salt tablets but made no effort to increase his water intake.

By the end of five days, Kevin was so weak he found it hard to exercise at all. As his fatigue increased, he mistakenly thought he wasn't getting enough salt and downed even more tablets.

I was called in by his parents who had noticed a change in Kevin's personality and didn't like the way he looked. He was running a 100° temperature.

I recognized that he was suffering from heat exhaustion. His symptoms: elevated temperature, extreme fatigue, muscle weakness, and a personality change. A blood test disclosed far too much salt in his blood.

Besides gulping down too many salt tablets, Kevin made other mistakes. He did too much too soon — not giving his body enough time to become accustomed to the heat. He worked out at the wrong time of the day, when temperatures were the hottest and the sun's rays were most direct.

Kevin stopped his do-it-yourself training program, drank lots of fruit juices, and threw away his salt tablets. Within three days, he was back on his feet, anxious to begin preseason football practice — this time under the supervision of a coach.

Weighing yourself daily can help you avoid Kevin's pitfalls. A sudden drop of a pound or two means you are not keeping up with your water loss.

Fruit juices will replace both the liquids lost in exercise and the potassium released from muscle cells into the bloodstream.

Other types of heat exhaustion

Heat exhaustion can also occur when the body has too little salt. Every year I treat athletes who have drunk large amounts of fluids and usually take extra salt all winter. As a result, their sweat glands and kidneys are unable to retain salt. In hot weather their salt requirements increase dramatically and they become salt deficient.

Simple dehydration takes place when an athlete sweats heavily. If he doesn't replace his fluid losses, he can develop heat exhaustion in a few hours even though he has a proper mineral balance.

The symptoms for both these types of heat exhaustion are similar: fatigue and weakness. Fever may be present with dehydration. The remedy for both is the same: Drink large amounts of fruit juices to replace potassium, and salt your food as your taste dictates.

Water Intoxication

If you notice you get a headache when you drink a lot of water, you may be susceptible to water intoxication, a condition characterized by headache and sometimes convulsions. This is what happens:

Normally you have the same concentrations of minerals inside and outside every cell of the body. When you drink large amounts of water, which has few minerals, the concentration of minerals outside the cells is lowered, while the mineral concentration inside the cells remains the same. This difference causes fluid to move into the cell. As a result, the brain cells swell well beyond their normal size, causing headache and even convulsions.

The remedy is to avoid drinking more than two glasses of water at one time unless you also eat something — an apple, a candy bar, or a sandwich. If you don't want to eat, drink mineral-rich fruit juices in place of water.

Heat Cramps

Because you sweat more in the summer, you are more likely to develop cramps due to diminished levels of minerals. Muscle cramps in the heat are the same as muscle cramps any other time. (See Chapter 10.)

They Didn't Drink

On July 19, 1977, a quarterback Billy Kilmer of the Washington Redskins and four of his pro football teammates were hospitalized with heat exhaustion suffered in the 100° F. temperature at their Carlisle, Pennsylvania, training camp.

All five, complaining of severe cramps, became ill after practice. All were victims of a dangerous, though less complex, form of heat exhaustion called simple dehydration with no change in the salt level of the blood.

By filling up on fruit juices, Kilmer and his teammates were back on the sweltering practice field the next day.

Training When Winter Is Worst

Provided that you understand the effects of cold weather and know how to prepare for them, exercising in the cold can be a safe, pleasant, and invigorating experience.

Here are the rules for cold weather exercise:

Dress adequately so that your clothes will help you retain body heat. Pay particular attention to protecting your fingers, ears, toes, and nose.

Eat heartily. It takes calories to keep you warm in cold weather.

To acclimatize to cold, you must train in the cold.

Know the progressive warning signs of hypothermia (a drop of one or more degrees in internal body temperature). These are: slurred speech, loss of coordination of the hands, inability to walk, and mental confusion.

Know the warning signs of impending frostbite — a burning and stinging of the skin, redness, numbness, and poor hand and foot coordination.

How Your Body Protects Itself against the Cold

A few years ago Dave Knighton, a marathon runner from Washington, D.C., and I were competing in a twenty-mile street race in a driving snowstorm. The wind-chill factor had dropped below zero. As we ran past skidding cars, Dave said with a smile, "Imagine those crazy drivers out here on a day like this!" The motorists probably thought we were the crazy ones.

While we were running in the race, we were comfortable and the cold didn't bother us. Our bodies were producing fifteen to twenty times as much heat as those of the people riding in the cars. Even joggers who creep along at a twelve-minute-mile pace increase their heat production almost tenfold. That's the reason that football players on the field do not suffer from the cold while you may be freezing in the stands. You can protect yourself to some extent, however, by jumping up and down.

To protect you from the effects of cold, your body makes use of the following responses and special structures:

Your brain sends out signals along nerves to close down the circulation to the skin. This conserves heat because it is

Cold-Weather Athletes

Tim Caldwell and Pete Patterson, both top skiers, are cold-weather performers. So are the Minnesota Vikings, the Buffalo Bills, the Green Bay Packers, and other National Football League teams from northern parts of the country.

Roy Hatch, one of the nation's best parachute jumpers, practices in the cold weather. He falls at speeds of 120 to 180 miles an hour and, at 32° F., exposes his body to a wind-chill factor of −40° F.

Jerry Martin, a distance runner who worked on the Alaskan pipeline at Prudhoe Bay in 1976, ran a mile when the wind-chill factor was 90° below zero (−68° C.). Afterward he said, "It was really cold that night. Mentally I was ready to do five miles. But running into the wind was laborious and cold." He suffered no ill effects.

Exercise Warms You

Parachutist Roy Hatch reports that he doesn't feel the cold in the 25 seconds of free fall.

"Maybe it is because I'm doing style turns in that time and I'm so busy concentrating that I don't think about the cold," he says.

The truth is that his body is producing more heat through exercise during that 25-second period. Hatch says he is bothered by cold on the plane ride up to 6,600-foot altitude and during the 1½ minutes it takes to reach the ground after the parachute is opened. During these two periods, Hatch is sedentary.

through the skin that heat is lost. If you continue to lose heat, your body then shuts down the blood supply to your arms and legs.

- You start to shiver—the body's response to a drop in temperature. Your muscles alternately contract and relax at a rapid pace. More than 60 percent of the energy produced by shivering gives off heat.
- You have fat under your skin which insulates your body from cold. Fat provides more than 50 percent of the body's insulation. Skin, fascia, and muscle provide the remaining 50 percent. That's why fit people with some fat handle cold weather better than those who are lean.
- Your arteries, which bring warm blood to the skin, lie next to veins, which bring cold blood from the skin. Thus, heat from the arteries warms the veins along their entire course back to the inner parts of the body. By the time cold blood from the skin reaches your internal organs, it has been significantly warmed.

Winter Running Tip

If you plan to jog or run for some distance, plot your course so you will run against the wind on the way out and with the wind on the way back. If you start running with the wind, the body will be warmer, produce more sweat, and your clothes will fill with perspiration. When you run against the wind, you will be colder, and your wet clothes will draw away your body heat.

What to Wear

Proper winter wear is a must.

Not only must you dress for the cold, you must also protect yourself from the wind because it can greatly increase the discomfort and danger of exposure to cold. A 35° F. day with a 40-mile-per-hour wind has the same effects as a 0° F. day. With certain severe combinations of temperature and wind, exposed flesh will freeze within one minute and irreversible damage occurs.

Wind-Chill Factors

WIND (MPH)	TEMPERATURE (FAHRENHEIT)																				
Calm	40°	35°	30°	25°	20°	15°	10°	5°	0°	−5°	−10°	−15°	−20°	−25°	−30°	−35°	−40°	−45°	−50°	−55°	−60°
											Equivalent Chill Temperature										
5	35°	30°	25°	20°	15°	10°	5°	0°	−5°	−10°	−15°	−20°	−25°	−30°	−35°	−40°	−45°	−50°	−55°	−65°	−70°
10	30°	20°	15°	10°	5°	0°	−10°	−15°	−20°	−25°	−35°	−40°	−45°	−50°	−60°	−65°	−70°	−75°	−80°	−90°	−95°
15	25°	15°	10°	0°	−5°	−10°	−20°	−25°	−30°	−40°	−45°	−50°	−60°	−65°	−70°	−80°	−85°	−90°	−100°	−105°	−110°
20	20°	10°	5°	0°	−10°	−15°	−25°	−30°	−35°	−45°	−50°	−60°	−65°	−75°	−80°	−85°	−95°	−105°	−110°	−115°	−120°
25	15°	10°	0°	−5°	−15°	−20°	−30°	−35°	−45°	−50°	−60°	−65°	−75°	−80°	−90°	−95°	−105°	−110°	−120°	−125°	−135°
30	10°	5°	0°	−10°	−20°	−25°	−30°	−40°	−50°	−55°	−65°	−70°	−80°	−85°	−95°	−100°	−105°	−115°	−120°	−130°	−140°
35	10°	5°	−5°	−10°	−20°	−25°	−35°	−40°	−50°	−60°	−65°	−75°	−80°	−90°	−100°	−105°	−115°	−120°	−130°	−135°	−145°
40*	10°	0°	−5°	−15°	−20°	−30°	−35°	−45°	−55°	−60°	−70°	−75°	−85°	−95°	−100°	−110°	−115°	−125°	−130°	−140°	−150°

Little danger   Increasing danger (Flesh may freeze within one minute)   Great danger (Flesh may freeze within 30 seconds)

*Winds above 40 mph have little additional effect.

Reprinted with permission from *Running with the Elements* published by the editors of *Runner's World Magazine*.

Covering the body

The amount and type of clothing you wear depends on your sport and the weather. Sports that require continuous exercise, such as cross-country skiing and running, do not require as much clothing as sports in which the exercise is frequently interrupted, such as downhill skiing, sledding, skating, and ski jumping. While participating in sports, your body produces heat continually — so much so that you sweat profusely. When you stop exercising, you will be covered with sweat and your heat output will decrease. As a result, you will feel cold. This happens commonly to downhill skiers, who generate a great deal of heat as they ski down the slopes. They feel cold when they stand around waiting for the ski lift to carry them back to the top.

In effect, skiers need two types of clothing: light clothing when they come down the slopes and well-insulated clothing to warm them while they are waiting for the ski lift. For this reason, all participants in stop-and-go sports should layer their clothing.

Multiple layers of clothing trap air between each layer, and air is one of the best insulators. Also, the outer layers of clothing can be added and discarded as needed.

As different materials have different insulating properties, some should be worn close to the skin while others should be used as an outside covering.

For example, because cotton absorbs sweat readily, it should be worn next to your body. By carrying the water away from your skin, it prevents evaporation and keeps your skin from cooling rapidly. For the same reason that cotton is such an excellent inside garment, it is the worst possible outside material. Because it absorbs water so readily, it loses almost all of its insulating properties when it becomes wet from rain or snow. Thus, blue jeans, which are made of cotton, when wet can drain away your body heat so fast that you will quickly begin to feel cold. The same applies to cotton sweat shirts and denim jackets. Even the finest goose-down jackets also become useless when wet. They too drain away body heat.

Wool is the best material for your outer layer of clothing. Even when it is wet, it will not draw away your body heat. Wool dries from the inside out. Thus, the dry inner part of a woolen jacket still maintains its insulating properties. You won't want to wear wool against your skin. Not only is it itchy, but it also won't carry the sweat away from your skin surface.

A windbreaker may also be worn, but many athletes

Dress Warmly

Tim Caldwell, the cross-country skier, can attest to this. In 1977, he did not dress warmly enough for a 50 kilometer pre-World Cup competition held in Finland in temperatures of $-20°$ F.

"Because I had on only a T-shirt and a running suit, I got cold on the down hills when the wind was blowing against my body," he recalls. "At thirty-nine kilometers I hit the wall — got dizzy and felt weak. My arms and legs wouldn't respond — just numbness.

"I finished the course, but I was not really conscious of what was happening in the last eleven kilometers."

won't use them because they block the passage of air and increase sweating.

The best material for the middle layer of clothing is down. It traps air so efficiently that as long as it is dry, it is the best insulating material pound for pound that is known to man. For these reasons, a down vest is an excellent investment.

Covering the extremities

Cold is felt first in the fingers, toes, and ears. That's why athletes or fitness enthusiasts can exercise with minimal clothing in moderately cold weather so long as they wear mittens, warm socks, and hats.

Mittens are superior to gloves because all the fingers warm each other in one compartment. Down is the preferred lining because it traps air. The circulating air also allows the mittens to dry between wearings, thus resisting molding.

A woolen cap that covers the ears protects the head best. In frigid weather a scarf or collar that can be raised to cover part of the face will be useful.

When you exercise, your feet generate a large amount of heat. As long as you keep them dry, shoes or ski boots and socks will be adequate protection.

What to Eat

It takes a great deal of food to supply the calories needed to heat your body in cold weather. More than 60 percent of the calories you burn end up heating your body. Less than 40 percent fuel your muscles. The harder you exercise, the more heat your body produces.

The best foods for fuel contain carbohydrates and fat. In cold-weather training, eat waffles, oatmeal, pancakes with butter and syrup, raisins, nuts, bread, and fruits.

What Not to Drink

Drinking large amounts of alcohol before going out into the cold, or while in it, can be extremely dangerous because it dulls the senses. A drunk person is not as sensitive to pain and doesn't get out of the cold when his skin starts to hurt.

Protecting the Extremities

Some competitive runners use old army socks as a kind of thumbless mitten to protect their hands. Skier Tim Caldwell wears handball gloves with wool or silk inserts.

Even though the free-fall part of his jump lasts only 25 seconds, parachutist Hatch says that any skin exposed to the air "really hurts, especially the nose, ears, and hands. My hands get so cold that I have problems grasping the toggles to guide the parachute down," he says. "After we jump, all of us stand on the ground and clap our hands so we can bend them again."

Many athletes won't cover their legs unless the wind-chill factor drops below 30 degrees; even then they wear only long johns and sweatpants.

Football star O. J. Simpson complains that too much clothing on his legs slows him down. He wears cutoff long johns on the upper part of his body, and rubs liniment on his legs when the temperature falls.

"I really can't bundle up, because I can't maneuver," says Simpson. "I have to cut out the knees of my long johns to get flexibility."

Frank Shorter won a National AAU Cross Country Championship in 20-degree temperature with his legs covered only by ladies' pantyhose.

Alcohol also widens the blood vessels in the skin and increases heat loss.

Acclimatizing to the Cold

Have you noticed that you're bothered more by freezing temperatures during the first few days of a skiing trip than you are after a couple of weeks? There's a logical explanation. Your body acclimatizes to the cold by producing more heat. One must exercise in the cold to become accustomed to the cold.

Scientists can measure this. On exposure to cold, the fingers of a person who has adjusted to cold have a greater blood supply and warmer temperature than those of one who has not adjusted.

Some mountain climbers prepare for the cold by taking progressively colder baths. This is nonsense! You can't exercise effectively sitting in a bathtub.

I know of skiers who ski without gloves to harden themselves against the cold. Although I admire their ability to suffer, the procedure is painful and I do not recommend it.

Cold-Weather Dangers

There are two dangerous cold-weather syndromes: frostbite, which occurs when the skin temperature drops below 32° F., and hypothermia, when the internal body temperature drops one or more degrees. Your can develop very low skin temperature and still have a normal body temperature. A normal body temperature of 98.6° F. has been maintained by English Channel swimmers while swimming for fifteen hours in water that had lowered their skin temperature to 59° F., a temperature 38 degrees lower than that of their bodies. However, in water temperature below 50° F., even these athletes cannot produce sufficient heat to maintain their body temperature for even a few minutes.

Predisposing Factors to Cold Injury

Subfreezing temperature
Increased wind velocity
Lack of adequate protective clothing
Wet clothing
Prolonged exposure to the cold
Fatigue
Injury
Dehydration
Poor nutrition
Contact with cold metals
Poor motivation
Ingestion of large amounts of alcohol

Frostbite

Frostbite is the condition in which body tissue is destroyed by freezing. Ice crystals form in the fluid around the cells and blood vessels freeze so that no blood can circulate. As the skin starts to freeze, it becomes so painful that the only people who ever develop serious cases of frostbite are those who are unable to get out of the cold: people who are unconscious, cross-country skiers who are lost, and mountain climbers who aren't able to return to camp before nightfall.

Causes

As your skin temperature drops from 98.6° F., the blood vessels in the skin close down and the skin appears white. Shut off from its blood supply, which is the source of its heat, the skin cools rapidly until it reaches 59° F. At this point the body attempts to save the skin by opening up its blood vessels and bringing warm blood to it. The skin appears red, feels warm, and a burning sensation begins, which develops into severe pain. As the skin continues to cool, it becomes numb and the pain disappears. When the skin temperature drops below freezing, circulation stops completely, the tissue freezes, and the skin develops a white, waxy appearance that feels like a frozen piece of meat.

Skin, blood vessels, and muscles are frozen first. As the temperature continues to drop, even the tendons and bones become frozen.

Treatment

Frostbite can be a serious condition and is best treated by a physician. Because the damage is less severe when the tissue is rapidly rewarmed, a physician will immerse the frostbitten arm or leg in water that is heated up to 108° F. This procedure may be extremely painful and may require narcotics. On thawing, the frostbitten area becomes bright red and a burning pain develops. In cases of bad frostbite the pain becomes increasingly severe and large, blood-filled blisters appear four to forty-eight hours later. In the next few weeks, the blisters lose their fluid and thick black scabs form over them. During the next two to six weeks, the scabs fall off and the skin attempts to heal. In the most severe cases, the skin does not heal and a finger or toe may be lost.

It is difficult for even the most experienced physicians to determine the severity of frostbite at the outset. The only differences between superficial and deep frostbite show up after the skin has thawed. As a rule, deep frostbite develops blisters within a few hours after thawing, while superficial frostbite develops them a day or two later. Deep frostbite is usually more painful, has much larger blisters and much more swelling, and often develops gangrene, a condition in which the skin dies, turns a dark black color, and then shrivels up and sloughs off.

Because gangrenous tissue has no blood supply to bring in the body's immune defenses, it is easily infected. If the signs of infection develop — red streaks, yellow pus, or fever — the physician will prescribe antibiotics. Infection in this tissue is extremely dangerous because it can spread through the body and cause death.

Once you have had frostbite, the blood vessels in the limbs may be irreparably damaged. As a result of this, pain, markedly increased sweating of previously injured skin, and a numb feeling may persist for years.

What you can do

Because your fingers and toes are the tissues most likely to develop frostbite, you should wear well-insulated mittens and boots. You should also cover your body. As your body starts to cool, the blood supply to the fingers and toes is shut down first, making them more susceptible to frostbite. Because almost 20 percent of your body heat can be lost through your head, you must also wear a warm hat that covers your ears.

You may get frostbite despite all your precautions, so be alert for its symptoms in yourself and others. The affected part looks white and hard, and feels numb. See a doctor right away. If this is impossible, rewarm the affected part rapidly in a warm-water bath. If the affected person is suffering solely from frostbite and has no heart or lung problems, Dr. William Mills, Jr., an orthopedic surgeon in Alaska and a consultant in cold injury to the Army Surgeon General, recommends rapid thawing at a temperature of 100° to 108° F. Under no circumstances should you allow the water temperature to exceed 112° F. Excessive heat — temperatures greater than 115° F. — gives absolutely disastrous results. *Furthermore, do not expose the frostbitten area to cold again* or attempt to thaw the frozen area while outdoors. Rewarming and refreezing a frostbitten area is far more dangerous than leaving the

How Napoleon Lost the War

During his war with Russia, Napoleon lost most of his army to frostbite. During the night, his soldiers would rewarm their frozen limbs. The next day they would go out and become frostbitten again, develop gangrene, and eventually lose their fingers and toes.

tissue frozen. Each successive freezing causes further damage to tissue that has already been damaged.

Hypothermia

On almost any Sunday afternoon in the winter, members of the Coney Island Polar Bears can be seen sunning themselves and swimming in the ice-cold water off Coney Island, New York. While onlookers may shudder sympathetically as the Polar Bears emerge from the water, the Polar Bears don't seem to have any problem with the cold.

Al Mottola, the president of the Bears, says: "When I get out of the water after a swim, I feel great. My skin is red all over, just like rubbing it briskly with a Turkish towel. I love that glowing feeling of my skin."

Why don't the Polar Bears get into trouble? Because they get out of the water quickly when their skin starts to turn red.

When the skin is exposed to cold, the body first attempts to conserve heat by closing down its blood vessels. This causes the skin to appear white. As the skin cools further to 59° F., the body tries to rewarm it by opening up the skin blood vessels. This causes the skin to turn red.

At this point, the body temperature starts to fall from 98.6° F., and a person must get out of the cold or he will develop hypothermia, which can *kill*.

In March 1968, eight marines and one sailor from the Quantico Marine Base in Virginia were paddling a canoe on the Potomac River when suddenly it tipped over. Although they were expert swimmers in superb physical condition and were less than one hundred feet from shore, they all died from hypothermia within minutes.

Why did they die? When they hit the cold water, their body temperatures dropped rapidly, which paralyzed their arms and legs. They were unable to swim and drowned. This will happen to everyone within a few minutes of immersion in water that has a temperature of 50° F. or less.

Here's what happens as your body temperature decreases:

a one-degree drop: Your speech becomes slurred.
a two-degree drop: Your fingers become clumsy, feel numb, and lose their strength. You start to shiver.

"Committing Suicide"

Swimming in winter can bring all kinds of attention. Al Mottola recalls a vacation in Northern Florida when it was so cold the motel pool had frozen.

"We were out cracking the ice in our bathing suits when the police rode up," he says. "They thought we were trying to commit suicide. We had to explain to them that winter swimming was our sport.

"The next day, the newspaper headlines read, 'Coney Island Polar Bears Invade Our Town.' We had a big write-up with our pictures featured on the front page."

a three-degree drop: Your feet lose their strength and you stumble and fall.

a four-degree drop: Your brain is affected and you have difficulty thinking clearly.

a nine-degree drop: Shivering is replaced by muscle rigidity.

a fourteen-degree drop: You lose consciousness and your heartbeat becomes irregular.

a twenty-three-degree drop: Death results from heart failure.

Whether you are a backpacker, a mountain climber, or a cross-country skier, you should be able to recognize the stages of hypothermia. Here's a story of a backpacker who did.

"On a backpacking trip on the Appalachian Trail, it started to rain. One of the ladies with us began to shiver and sat down on a tree stump. Her speech became slurred and she told us that she was very tired. After a few minutes she was unable to stand up. That meant that her body temperature had dropped below 95° F. We immediately set up a tent, took off her wet clothes, and had several of the other women climb into a sleeping bag with her. Their body heat warmed her and within ten minutes she felt better. After another half hour it had stopped raining, and we headed back to the lodge."

When your clothes are wet, they act as a wick to carry away your body heat.

The treatment of hypothermia is rapid rewarming. If you have a warm bath available, heat it to body temperature and place the victim in it. If a bath is not available, put the victim under the covers with a warming device, whether it is a couple of hot water bottles or another human body. If you are alone and develop any of the signs of hypothermia, get yourself dry as soon as possible and cover yourself with several blankets.

13.

Sex and Sports

In a computer search of the medical literature gathered over the last twenty years by the National Library of Medicine, I couldn't find a single well-controlled study on the relationship between fitness and sexual performance.

To get some answers, I conducted many personal interviews with athletes, fitness enthusiasts, and leading medical authorities. I also asked the readers of *Running Times* to answer a questionnaire on the subject.

From these different sources, I came to this conclusion: The old adage that sex and athletics don't mix is untrue. On the contrary, athletes have better sex lives.

How Exercise Affects Sex

I believe that when you are fit, you are a better sex partner and tend to enjoy sex more. Dr. William Masters, a leading authority on sex, points out that there is no specific proof for this belief, but he says: "A person who has good physical fitness invariably functions more effectively sexually than a person in poor shape. Sexual function is a physiologic process and every physiologic process works better in a good state of general health than in a poor one."

If you are in poor shape, a well-planned fitness program may improve your sexual performance.

Fit for Bed

The more fit I am for road racing, the more fit I am for sexual activities. Running allows me to have greater stamina in bed.
  — *A 27-year-old male physical therapist*

. . . But There Are Limits

An 85-mile week combined with a 10-hour working day leaves me barely enough energy to crawl from the dinner table to the bed. My non-marathon-running wife has a rule of thumb — 15 miles or more per day renders me sexually useless.
— *A 43-year-old marathon runner who works for the Department of Defense*

Making love, like exercise, increases your body's requirements for oxygen and nutrition. To meet this need, your heart must pump increased amounts of blood. Heart rates as high as 180 beats per minute have been recorded during sexual relations.

"In general, participation in sexual relations doesn't require any more energy than walking up a flight of stairs, or running a forty-yard dash," says Dr. Masters.

There are some people, however, who are in such poor physical shape that they cannot walk up a flight of stairs without becoming breathless, or run forty yards. During lovemaking, these individuals often become short of breath and their muscles become tired. They must slow down and stop. Many times, this leads to disappointment and anxiety.

The ideal love act happens when both partners stimulate each other with ever-increasing intensity until climax. According to our survey, individuals who are fit don't tire easily during lovemaking and can participate in sexual relations more intensely and for a longer period of time. They find this satisfying and rewarding.

Indeed, in response to our survey on the sexual habits of athletes, one runner sent us a bumper sticker that says: "Marathon runners keep it up longer." Although there's no scientific evidence to substantiate this, virtually every male and female marathoner we interviewed agrees with the sticker.

Dr. Joan Ullyot, a competitive marathon runner and author of the book *Women's Running,* told me: "After talking with women marathon runners from all over the country, I can tell you that they take advantage of their increased endurance in making love."

When one partner is fit and the other isn't, it leads to a sexual imbalance. A woman runner who is married to a champion marathoner says, "There is no way that a nonexerciser can keep up in bed with a person in shape. Most of the wives of marathon runners in our group are runners. They feel that running improves sexual stamina."

People who are fit look good and feel proud of their bodies. They don't have sagging stomachs, pendulous hips, and double chins. They are usually not inhibited about their bodies and are more sure of themselves. Because they usually take a more active part in sexual relations, they tend to be better partners.

Fit for Fun

I feel that sexual relations have improved since I started to run. My husband and I are happier doing things together and this reflects itself in our desire to have sex together. The intensity of my feelings during the love act have definitely increased since I have been running.
— *A 36-year-old female schoolteacher who is married to a marathon runner and who recently took up running*

How Sex Affects Athletic Performance

We found general agreement that sexual relations on the night before competition does not impair athletic performance and may even improve it.

Professional athletes almost unanimously told me that sexual relations the night before games were beneficial. In fact, we found many coaches who actually encourage it.

Weeb Ewbank, former coach of the New York Jets, used to say: "Players should relax before competition. If they feel that sex before a game is relaxing, we encourage it."

"Having successful sex before competition has many pluses," says Olympic track coach Brooks Johnson. "It can be relaxing and fulfilling. For some athletes, it has the same effect as having a good rubdown."

The myth that sexual relations impair athletic performance probably started with the Old Testament. It cautioned warriors not to go to battle immediately after marriage and said neighbors should help a newlywed with his chores so that he could adjust to the joys of matrimony.

The American Medical Association's Committee on the Medical Aspects of Sports reports that sexual relations on the night before a game do not hinder athletic performance provided that sex is a regular part of the athlete's life.

The only ways that sexual relations on the night before competition can have a detrimental effect on the athlete's performance are:

> If the athlete believes that it will impair his or her athletic performance.
> If the athlete doesn't get enough sleep.

Donald L. Cooper, team physician for Oklahoma State University, says: "Most team physicians that I have visited feel that a normal pattern of sexual practice is not detrimental as long as a proper amount of sleep is obtained."

Casey Stengel, the late skipper of the New York Yankees, put it pithily: "It isn't sex that wrecks these guys, it's staying up all night looking for it."

I once believed that sex the night before competition would hurt my performance. Because I cut back on my training mileage three days before a race, I had extra energy and no place to spend it. On pre-race nights, I often couldn't sleep. On the morning of the race, I would wake up exhausted.

After I had been competing for several years, I succumbed one night to desire, and the next day I ran a superb race. I've learned since then that sexual relations on the night prior to a race actually improves my performance.

We found only one case of a married professional athlete who abstained from sexual relations on the night before a game. Says his National Basketball Association coach: "His college coach told him, 'Don't do it before a game. Your jump shot might fall two feet short.'

"I talked to the team doctor about him. The doctor said that was the reason the guy was so uptight before a game."

While there is general agreement among athletes, coaches, trainers, and physicians that on the night before competition athletes can engage in sexual relations without harming their performance, there is disagreement whether they can safely participate just before competition.

Dr. Masters says: "Restricting a player from sexual relations before a game is hogwash. Pre-game warm-ups use far more energy than sexual relations."

Dr. George Sheehan, a father of twelve, says, "My personal experience has convinced me that peak performance in middle- and long-distance races is possible within hours of sexual activity."

Dr. Craig Sharp, Britain's chief medical adviser at the 1972 Olympics, cites two cases of runners who performed outstanding feats on the track shortly after sexual relations. One, a middle-distance Olympic runner, set a world record an hour after making love. The other, a British miler, ran a four-minute mile.

A forty-year-old male runner who answered the *Running Times* questionnaire says: "For the last year, I've been conducting what Dr. Sheehan would call an experiment of one. I run in races almost every weekend, and half the time my wife and I made love the morning of the race, anywhere from one to four hours before the start of competition. It doesn't help my time, and it doesn't seem to hurt it."

One hockey player who holds superstar status says that he normally has sexual relations four hours before the face-off.

We did find a few athletes who felt their performance was hindered by sexual relations just before competition. "I remember one Sunday afternoon, I had sex a few hours before game time," recalls a hockey superstar. "My legs were so rubbery that I didn't know what I was doing out on

Hurt by What They Believe

Some of the New York Yankees starting pitchers believe in the "strength-sapping" power of sex and many of them will forgo sex on the day they pitch.

Helped by What He Believes

I am well aware of a world-class sprinter who, one-half hour after masturbating, went out and set a world's record.

— WILLIAM MASTERS, M.D.,
world-famous expert on sexual relations

the ice. It was the worst game of my career. There is no way that you can recover two hours after making love."

"When I run shortly after sexual relations," reports a top marathon runner, "my legs are heavy and my times are slower. I tried a running experiment. I ran twenty miles over the same course every Sunday. The runs immediately after sex averaged 2 hours and 16 minutes. The times without sex averaged 2 hours and 10 minutes. As a result, I've given up Sunday morning sex."

Based on our survey and interviews, I've concluded that athletes have more fulfilling sex lives. For the majority of Americans, sports and sex are similar in that everyone can participate, and it's more important to take part than to sit on the sidelines.

14.

Why and How to Choose a Sportsmedicine Physician

Diagnosis of Disease in Athletes Requires Special Knowledge

There are good reasons why you should seek a sportsmedicine physician for the treatment of a sports injury.

Active people are physically and emotionally different from sedentary ones.

Most physicians have not had special training in sportsmedicine. Consequently, even outstanding physicians who don't treat athletes regularly often make mistakes in the diagnosis and treatment of athletes' medical problems.

Many physicians are not yet aware that athletes are so supernormal that they have their own set of normal values for laboratory tests. What could be interpreted as abnormal in sedentary people may often be normal in athletes. Because physicians may be misled by these laboratory tests and diagnose diseases that are not present, we call them "pseudodiseases." Here are some examples:

"Anemia"

In 1968, Brooks Johnson brought Olympian Ester Stroy to me to evaluate her for fatigue. A routine blood test showed that she had anemia — a low concentration of red blood cells.

I remember telling Brooks, "If she can make the Olympic team with anemia, imagine what she could do if her blood level were normal."

Then I tested other members of Brooks's Sports International Team and was amazed to find that most of the girls were anemic. Because I thought that the girls were not eating properly, I gave them vitamin tablets with iron. I was surprised when the supplements did not raise their hemoglobin levels.

Puzzled, I went to the medical library at the National Institutes of Health and found that athletes have an increased blood volume. Thus, even though athletes may have normal or increased amounts of red blood cells in their bodies, their increased blood volume lowers the concentration of those cells and they appear to be anemic.

Over the years I have seen many other cases of laboratory tests that would be abnormal in nonathletes and normal in athletes.

"Liver disease"

"How could I have hepatitis when I ran a marathon three days ago?" asked Colonel Ken Baker of Arlington, Virginia. At a routine physical examination at the Pentagon, his blood test showed an elevated enzyme level commonly associated with hepatitis.

Marathoner Ed Barron, president of the Potomac Valley Seniors Running Club in the Washington, D.C., area, had a similar experience. As a result of elevated enzymes in his bloodstream, he was hospitalized for a suspected liver tumor. Because every other liver test was normal, his physician was puzzled.

Almost all athletes have elevated enzyme levels after competition. During heavy exercise, the muscles are slightly damaged and release enzymes into the bloodstream. In liver disease, the damaged liver cells release similar enzymes. The similarity of the two conditions often confuses physicians who are not experienced in the treatment of athletes.

If you are found to have elevated blood enzyme levels, don't panic. Wait forty-eight hours and repeat the tests. By that time, the enzyme levels should have returned to normal. If your blood tests are still abnormal, you need a more detailed medical evaluation.

Why and How to Choose a Sportsmedicine Physician | 173

"Kidney disease"

A top high school cross-country runner was referred to me because his regular physician had found red blood cells in his urine.

In nonathletes, bloody urine can signal serious diseases — kidney stones, bladder and kidney infection, tumors (including cancer), and other diseases.

I asked the athlete to bring me a fresh urine specimen voided in the morning before exercise. Because it was normal, I told him to continue running. If that specimen had contained red blood cells, I would have recommended an extensive medical evaluation.

As early as 1894, Dr. L. Dickinson reported to the Clinical Society of London that athletes often develop bloody urine after hard exercise. Medical scientists don't know why the red blood cells appear in the urine. It may be that when the kidneys are shaken during exercise, red blood cells pass through the glomerulus, the kidney filter, which under normal conditions has pores that are too small to let the cells pass. Another recent theory is that the red blood cells come from shaking the bladder when it is stretched with urine.

Usually blood in the urine can be seen only with the aid of a microscope. But bright-red urine occurs in athletes and is not a reason to hit the panic button. Your urine should be free of blood forty-eight hours after you stop exercising. If it is not, further medical evaluation is indicated. Red blood cells are not the only cause of red urine. Other causes are:

Hemoglobin, the pigment released into the bloodstream when red blood cells burst during very hard exercise

Myoglobin, the red pigment released from muscles when they are damaged; low-carbohydrate diets and dehydration may increase the likelihood of this happening

Pigments in the diet from foods such as beets or certain antibiotics

Besides red blood cells, post-exercise urine can contain protein and cell deposits, both of which are usually absent in the urine of healthy persons. If the urine still contains any of these elements forty-eight hours after the athlete stops exercising, he or she should have a thorough medical evaluation.

"Infection"

Mike Frary went to his doctor because he felt tired. He had previously run one hundred miles a week and now had trouble running forty. His muscles ached constantly, he had difficulty sleeping at night, and everything his wife said irritated him.

His physician ordered blood tests, which revealed a higher than normal white blood cell count, often an indicator of infection. His physician prescribed antibiotics. After two weeks of medication, he did not improve. Repeated blood tests showed that Frary's white blood cell count was still elevated.

At that point, Mike consulted me. After taking his history, I diagnosed his problem — the overtraining syndrome. (See Chapter 4.) Elevated white blood cell counts are common in people who overtrain.

I recommended that he stop training. Three weeks later, his white blood cell count returned to normal. His irascibility diminished, and he was eager to train again.

"Heart disease"

Electrocardiograms performed on normal, healthy athletes are often interpreted as abnormal. There are two reasons:

> The hearts of athletes beat irregularly more frequently than those of the general population. In the vast majority of cases, these irregular heart beats are not harmful.
>
> An electrocardiogram often cannot differentiate between the healthy, thick muscular wall of the athlete's heart and the thin, stretched, or damaged muscle of a person likely to have a heart attack.

Gaston Roelants, an Olympic champion distance runner, has an "abnormal" electrocardiogram. Kerry O'Brien, while the world record holder in the steeplechase, was told to stop running because of an "abnormal" electrocardiogram. Twenty-five percent of all runners over forty years of age have "irregular" electrocardiograms.

Dr. George Sheehan, a world-famous heart specialist who treats athletes, explains: "An athlete who submits to a routine electrocardiogram is playing Russian Roulette with his future. He has one chance in six of having an electrocardiogram that will bar him from competition. Black athletes should regard the electrocardiogram as their mortal enemy, as they have a higher incidence of 'abnormal' electrocardiograms."

Treatment of Injuries in Athletes Requires Special Knowledge

Many physicians are not aware that injuries to athletes often require treatments different from those for nonathletes. Furthermore, some therapies that produce good results in nonathletes may have a detrimental effect on athletes.

Take the case of a sixteen-year-old high school halfback who submits to a third painful steroid injection in his Achilles tendon. In his next scrimmage, he tears the tendon from his heel and is still limping a year later.

Because nonexercisers generally rest when they are injured, they can usually get away with steroid injections. But athletes and fitness buffs usually will not rest and may end up with serious complications. Dr. James Nicholas, one of the leading experts in sportsmedicine, warns: "The injection of steroids into tendons of athletes should be restricted."

The injections reduce the swelling and relieve pain. But as Dr. Mal Olix and Lou Unverforth of Ohio State Medical School have shown, they also weaken the tendons.

Dr. Don O'Donoghue explains why: "Tendons don't have much of a blood supply. If you put steroids into the tendon, the blood supply is shut off and the tissue dies. Then the athlete goes out and tears off the tendon."

A sportsmedicine physician should instruct the injured athlete to participate temporarily in a sport that rests his injured part but maintains his conditioning. Al Cantello, the cross-country coach at the United States Naval Academy, understands this sportsmedicine principle. In 1977, Tom MacNeil, one of the top runners at the Academy, broke a bone in his foot. Most physicians would have ordered him to rest and MacNeil would have lost most of his conditioning.

But not coach Cantello. On days when members of the team would go out on long runs, Cantello instructed MacNeil to ride a bicycle three times as far. On days when the team ran intervals, MacNeil swam them. By the end of the season, Tom MacNeil was still one of the top runners on the team.

Casts are another example of why exercisers should be treated differently. Although physicians apply casts routinely to nonathletes, they must avoid applying them to athletes for any length of time, if at all possible. Immobilizing muscles with a cast for as little as one week can cause them to weaken and become smaller. It may take a month of corrective exercise for the muscles to regain their strength.

To treat athletic injuries properly, physicians must understand the following factors that cause them and correct them where possible:

Poor training methods
Structural abnormalities that predispose you to injury
Trauma
Poor eating habits
Extremes in weather

These are discussed in detail in chapters 4, 6, 9, 10, 11, and 12.

How You Can Find a Sportsmedicine Physician

Because very few physicians treat athletic injuries on a full-time basis presently, you will have difficulty finding an experienced sportsmedicine physician. Most athletic problems are handled by an estimated 30,000 physicians who practice sportsmedicine on a part-time basis.

Allan J. Ryan, the editor of *The Physician and Sportsmedicine*, the most prestigious sportsmedicine journal in the country, says: "There are very few medical schools or residencies which offer training in sportsmedicine. Without courses, there is no way that you could give an examination to certify special competence in the field. Thus, sportsmedicine is not a recognized specialty such as internal medicine or pediatrics."

The Physician and Sportsmedicine has twenty-one physicians on its editorial board and not a single one lists sportsmedicine as his or her specialty.

Dr. Ryan continues: "There's an amateur tradition that goes along with sportsmedicine. Physicians give their services to athletes because of their own personal interest in them. Most sports injuries occur in high school athletes who don't have any financial independence. They must depend on their parents for support. As a result, most physicians couldn't afford to advertise that they treat only athletic injuries."

Most athletes and fitness buffs come to me because they

have been recommended by other athletes or because they know that I am an athlete.

I recommend that you try to find a physician who is also an athlete. He or she has probably seen similar problems or even had them.

If you live in a city with a college or professional team, call its trainer. He usually will recommend a physician experienced in the treatment of athletic injuries. If you live in a small town, call the high school coach.

If you still can't find a physician to treat your athletic injury, contact your regular physician. Often he will know the physicians in your community who specialize in treating athletes.

If he can't help, get in touch with the nearest medical school. Usually, they will refer you to their department of orthopedics. Invariably, they will have a physician who is experienced in treating athletic injuries.

If there is no medical school in your area, look in your phone book to find the address of your local medical society. Most of the counties in your state will have societies.

The American Medical Association is affiliated with medical societies in every state. If you can't find a local medical society, send a stamped, self-addressed envelope to:

American Medical Association
535 North Dearborn Street
Chicago, Illinois 60610

They will send you the name of the medical society closest to you.

After you have found your local medical society, call them and ask for the names of physicians who specialize in athletic injuries. If they are unable to name a specific physician, ask for the name of an orthopedist.

If you still have trouble finding a doctor, check the list of over two hundred members of the American Orthopaedic Society for Sports Medicine in Appendix A in the back of this book.

All traumatic injuries, such as those caused by a jarring tackle, falling, or stepping in a hole, are usually treated by a sportsmedicine orthopedist. However, wear and tear injuries of the lower extremity are usually treated by a sportsmedicine podiatrist or any other physician who is trained in biomechanics, the study of the structural balances of the body. You will find a list of members of the

American Academy of Podiatric Sports Medicine in Appendix B in the back of the book. If you can't find the name of a sportsmedicine podiatrist who practices near where you live, look for the name of a podiatrist in your local telephone book or call your local podiatry association.

If you're a skier, seek medical treatment where you are injured. Physicians who practice in ski areas generally have more experience with ski injuries than those who are situated elsewhere.

If you can't find a physician, find an athlete. He or she may be able to tell you where to locate help. You may also want to contact local or national athletic groups and find out what physicians they consult. For example, if you're a runner, contact the Road Runners Club of America, which has more than one hundred and fifty chapters nationally. To find the chapter closest to you, send a stamped, self-addressed envelope to:

Ellen Wessel, Director of Public Relations
Road Runners Club of America
1111 Army Navy Drive
Arlington, Virginia 22202

You can then contact the local chapter for the name of a physician who treats running injuries. You could also send a stamped, self-addressed envelope to:

National Jogging Association
1910 K Street, N.W.
Washington, D.C. 20006

I wrote letters to athletic associations throughout the country. As a rule, they do not keep lists of physicians and do not have enough personnel to answer queries about how to find them.

15.

Start Exercising Today!
A Step-by-Step Running Program

Besides contributing to better health and a longer lifespan, regular exercise can improve the quality of your life. It can decrease anxiety and alleviate depression, help you sleep soundly, add to your ability to concentrate and work, increase your stamina during lovemaking, and help you to lose weight.

With all these benefits, you should be either a confirmed exerciser or a participant in a sport you enjoy. You could attend a Yoga class, take aerobic dancing at your local YMCA, or play tennis or golf. But the sport that gives you the most exercise in the least amount of time is running. You don't need a partner. It's inexpensive and the only equipment you need is a good pair of running shoes. There's no waiting in line, and you can begin and end at your doorstep. I've run for many years and attribute much of my success in life to it. Without running, I wouldn't have the energy and stamina to work fourteen to sixteen hours a day.

The Difference between Running and Jogging

I consider myself a runner, not a jogger — and there is a major difference. A jogger jogs because he feels it will protect or improve his health. A runner runs even if he thinks it might kill him.

Physical Fitness

Seven medical experts were asked by the President's Council on Physical Fitness and Sports to rate fourteen sports and exercises on a scale of 0 to 3, indicating their effectiveness in promoting fitness. Thus, a rating of 21 for an exercise means that it was viewed as most beneficial, since each of the experts gave it a score of 3.

	STAMINA	MUSCULAR ENDURANCE	MUSCULAR STRENGTH	FLEXIBILITY	BALANCE	TOTAL
Handball/Squash	19	18	15	16	17	85
Jogging	21	20	17	9	17	84
Skiing — Downhill	16	18	15	14	21	84
Skating (ice or roller)	18	17	15	13	20	83
Skiing — Cross Country	19	19	15	14	16	83
Swimming	21	20	14	15	12	82
Bicycling	19	18	16	9	18	80
Basketball	19	17	15	13	16	80
Tennis	16	16	14	14	16	76
Calisthenics	10	13	16	19	15	73
Walking	13	14	11	7	8	53
Golf	8	8	9	8	8	41
Softball	6	8	7	9	7	37
Bowling	5	5	5	7	6	28

SOURCE: The President's Council on Physical Fitness and Sports.

Bill Emmerton, the professional marathoner who once ran through Death Valley, was asked what he would do if he were told that running might kill him. His answer: "I would go out and run ten miles. Can you think of a better way to die?"

Joggers and runners also train differently. Joggers almost never run fast enough to increase their pulse and breathing rates markedly, but runners run hard at least two or three times a week. To train your heart, you must increase your pulse rate.

If you can walk, you can jog. If you can jog, you can run. There is no age or sex barrier. If you want to do it, you can. But don't expect too much too soon. As I tell my students at the University of Maryland: "It takes many years to get out of shape. Don't think you can become fit in a week."

If you are more than thirty years old, I recommend a stress electrocardiogram — done while you exercise. The traditional electrocardiogram, taken while lying down, is not as valuable. A list of places where you can obtain a stress electrocardiogram is given in Appendix C.

If normal, the stress test will reassure you that an exercise-induced heart attack is remote. If the electrocardiogram is abnormal or you have a history of heart disease, your program should be supervised by a physician.

I must emphasize that on extremely rare occasions even fit runners have died while they are running. If you have any questions before or after you start the program, always check with your physician.

What to Wear

Shoes

The most important equipment you will buy are your shoes. Here's how to chose the right pair.

Make sure that the shoes fit. When you go to a shoe store, always have the length and width of your feet measured. If you are a D width, you can use any one of a number of excellent running shoes. However, if you are not a D width, insist that you be given a shoe with your specific width.

Many stores do not carry widths because they do not want to tie up their money by stocking extra shoes. Don't deal with these stores. They are likely to try to sell you shoes that do not fit your feet. As a result, you will develop blisters, corns, calluses, and pain in your feet.

New Balance and Brooks are examples of excellent running shoes that come in variable widths. Many of the other manufacturers have resisted making their shoes with variable widths. Only by refusing to buy shoes that don't fit will you force them to carry more sizes.

To gauge the proper length, make sure that there is a space the width of your thumb between the tip of your big toe and the front end of the shoe.

Be sure to get a shoe with all of the following features:

> A flexible sole. Bend the shoe. If the sole does not bend easily, when you wear it, you will be forced to exert extra pressure with each step. This causes injuries to the fascia on the bottom of your foot and your Achilles tendon.
> A pad under your arch. To limit pronation, your shoe should have a soft arch support built into the shoe.
> Flared heel, padded collar, stiff Achilles counter, and firm saddle. (See Chapter 11.) These features limit pronation.

The Great Demar

"Go, Clarence, go!" Boston fans cried as Clarence Demar, a small gray-haired man in his early sixties, ran through the city street.

To the working class of downtown Boston, Demar, winner of seven Boston Marathons, was a local hero. He was employed as a proofreader at the *Boston Globe*.

While growing up in Boston, I worked after school in a downtown delicatessen and often saw Demar running through the streets.

In 1953, my last year at Boston Latin High School, I saw Demar run the Boston Marathon. As he passed by, the crowds gave him a bigger ovation than the leaders of the race. For many spectators, the race was over after Demar ran by.

I was so awed by the great Demar that I wanted to emulate him. As a college freshman, I entered the Boston Marathon even though I knew very little about training for long runs. I hadn't run a single practice run of more than six miles and my legs went limp at twenty miles.

Suddenly, I heard a wild ovation from the huge crowd. Naively, I thought they were impressed by my Harvard jersey. Then I turned around and saw the legendary Demar, ringed by twenty-five runners.

He finished the race ten minutes ahead of me.

Even though Demar had a cancerous colon removed and had a colostomy, he continued to run. Just prior to his death, he competed in a ten-mile run in New Hampshire.

— GABE MIRKIN, M.D.

Socks

Wear thin stretch socks. Thick socks keep your shoes from fitting snugly and allow the feet to move in the shoe. This prevents the shoe from performing its major function — limiting pronation — and makes you more susceptible to injury.

Shorts

The major problem with many shorts is that they have a thick seam that rubs against the inner part of your thighs and causes an abrasion of the skin. To avoid this, always buy shorts that have a thin seam.

Nylon pants are superior to cotton. When they are wet, they dry almost immediately. They weigh less and don't tend to irritate as much as cotton.

Sweat suits

I prefer a suit that is made of a combination of cotton and an artificial material such as nylon or dacron. They last longer and feel better. Make sure that your suit has a pocket to hold money, keys, etc.

Hats

Always cover your head when the sun is out. Direct sunlight can make you tired as well as damage your skin. In very hot weather, you can use the hat as a receptacle for the water you pour on your head. A hot-weather hat should have a brim to keep the sun off your face and be made of a mesh material so that your sweat can evaporate through it.

In cold weather, always wear a hat that pulls down over your ears. Regular ski hats are ideal. In very cold weather, you may want to wear a skicap with a face mask.

Mittens

Always wear mittens in cold weather. Your fingers are more sensitive to cold than any other part of your body. Many runners use socks as a sort of thumbless mitten. They tell me that because the socks are lighter than regular mittens, they will not slow them down.

Why are mittens better than gloves? Each finger warms

another in a common chamber. Feather mittens are ideal: they are light and are good insulators.

The Pre-training Program

Here's a pre-training program to teach beginners how to start a running program. Dr. Roy Lindgren and I worked it up for the Montgomery County Health Department in Maryland. (If you can already jog ten minutes daily without stopping, you can skip the three steps that follow.)

Step 1. Start walking daily. Gradually increase the tempo until you are able to walk briskly for ten minutes a day. It's all right to walk so vigorously that you have to breathe deeply.

Step 2. Jog a few steps then walk a few steps. Do this for ten minutes each day. Be careful not to push yourself beyond mild breathlessness. Gradually decrease the walking and increase the jogging until you can jog continuously for ten minutes. Distance and speed are not important.

If you are in poor shape, it may take weeks or even months to achieve this level of fitness. But don't become impatient. Years of neglect can't be cured with a few weeks of exercise. For one of my patients, it took more than eight months to be able to jog continually for ten minutes. He first had to lose more than forty pounds and rehabilitate a heart and lungs that were damaged by twenty years of smoking. After three years in the program, he finished a marathon in under four hours.

Step 3. Jog daily for ten minutes for several weeks. Don't worry about distance or speed. Ten minutes of jogging is the minimum amount of time needed to condition you.

How to Run

Now you can begin training in earnest.

For an estimated 16.5 million Americans, jogging or running is the passport to physical fitness. But to get all the health-giving benefits from the running, you should become more than a jogger.

Jogging increases the pulse rate only a few beats per

Many Well-Known Americans Are Joining the Running Craze

Actress Brenda Vaccaro says, "I like to jog because it helps my love life."

"I expect to be jogging till I'm ninety," declared South Carolina Senator Strom Thurmond. At seventy-five, he looks as if he could.

Reporter–TV host Tom Brokaw says, "I feel guilty if I miss a single day."

Baritone Robert Merrill of the Metropolitan Opera memorizes lyrics as he jogs near his Westchester home.

Actress Shirley MacLaine, at age forty-two, runs 35 miles a week for weight control. After gaining 35 pounds on the McGovern-For-President, chicken-a-la-king circuit, she took up running to slim down.

John Archer, the vice president of the Joseph Schlitz Brewing Company, took up running at age forty-nine for therapy for a back injury he developed splitting firewood. He's now a marathoner.

minute and doesn't adequately stress the cardiovascular system. In preventing heart attacks and strengthening the heart muscle, it is less valuable than hard running. To get maximum benefit, you must run hard enough to raise your pulse rate to 120 beats per minute two or three times a week.

Proper running form is also important. A novice runner commonly makes two mistakes: landing on his toes and leaning forward. Toe running doesn't help you to run faster and doesn't increase your endurance. Instead, by straining your shin and calf muscles and your Achilles tendon, it increases your chances for foot and leg injuries, slows you down, and tires you more quickly.

Leaning forward shortens your stride and, by forcing you to resist the tendency to fall, will waste your energy. Bill Bowerman, the premier distance running coach in America, says: "Lean forward when you run only if you are trying to knock down a wall with your head."

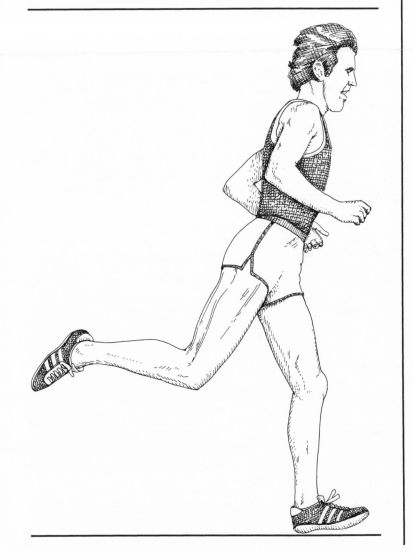

Proper Running Form

1) *Land on heel*
2) *Back straight*
3) *Elbows relaxed*
4) *Shoulders low*
5) *Hands loosely cupped*

Relax your elbows and let your arms swing freely. Your hands should be held at your belt line, and your fingers should be cupped loosely.

Your shoulders should be relaxed, with your head and your eyes forward.

Run with a short stride. Overstriding is a common mistake for high school runners and novices. When you do this, your body is not over your feet and you waste energy and tire more quickly.

Whether you are an 89-pound grandmother just starting a jogging program or an Olympic champion, the training rules are the same. Perhaps the most important rule of all: AVOID using the same training regimen day after day. It is ridiculous to run the same distance at the same pace day after day.

Building fitness means putting stress on the muscles, the heart, and the lungs — and then allowing sufficient time for the body to recover. After recovery, the body is stronger than before. This is called the overload principle and is based on the work of Hans Selye, a Canadian scientist.

Jack Schiff, a friend from Rockville, Maryland, recently confided that even though he's been running for years, he couldn't run more than five miles without stopping. I told him that any motivated individual can run a marathon. He looked at me in disbelief and asked: "What's wrong with me?"

Like most novice or unsupervised runners, Jack was running the same distance at the same pace day after day. Schiff wouldn't quit, but other runners, if they don't improve, give up. Some try to run as far as they can day after day. Injury or exhaustion often occurs and the result is always the same: a short-lived running program.

On the other hand, Dave Weiss of Silver Spring, Maryland, a weekend jogger who had never run over five miles, went to a seminar I presented to the District of Columbia Road Runners Club. Eight months later, he wrote me:

"You were so convinced that anyone could run a marathon that I believed you. Yesterday, I ran the Marine Corps Marathon in three hours and 27 minutes. I plan to run many more."

My Rules for Running

1. Don't run hard more than three times a week

To get a training effect, the heart rate must be increased to at least 60 percent of its maximum. Most physiologists recommend more than that: 160 beats per minute for the trained athlete and more than 120 for the casual athlete. However, because their leg muscles break down when they run hard every day, athletes also plan easy days on which they keep their pulses below that level.

Do not try to count your pulse. It will take some of the fun out of running. You can tell when your pulse rate is more than 120 because, at that pace, you will breathe deeply. It's called "sighing respiration" and makes talking difficult. I want to emphasize that you should not run so fast that you are gasping for air. That will only limit the distance you can run and increase your chances for injury. On the other hand, when you run on easy days, you should not be breathing hard. If you can't talk, you're running too fast.

You will improve from the stress applied on your hard days and recover faster by jogging at a relaxed pace on your easy days. If you skip an easy day, don't feel guilty. It's the hard days that will give you strength and endurance.

2. Don't run hard on consecutive days

When you exercise your muscles intensely, muscle cells are damaged, releasing enzymes into the bloodstream. The degree of damage can be measured by the level of these enzymes in your blood. Healing usually takes forty-eight hours and the muscles are stronger than before they were stressed.

Potassium — given off from the muscles to prevent overheating — and glycogen — the main fuel of muscular exercise — are used up and must be replaced. Depending on how hard you have exercised, recovery can take from ten hours to ten full days.

3. Once a week, run until your muscles ache

For a beginner, it may take a mile; for some marathoners, up to thirty miles.

Muscle pain may indicate that you are running out of glycogen — and this is good. The more often you deplete

---

Running Hints

If you must run on the street, always run against traffic. That way you can always see a runner's worst enemy — the car.

Dr. Ernst Van Aaken, a world-famous sportsmedicine physician, was hit from behind by an automobile and lost both legs at age sixty-two.

If you must run at night, wear white clothing or reflectors or carry a flashlight.

Don't run on a track. It's boring. The scenery never changes. If you must run on a track, change directions frequently. Otherwise, you may stress one leg more than the other and develop an injury.

If a dog nips at your heels, do not appear frightened. Move out of the dog's territory by crossing the street. If he follows you, stare him in the eyes, and let out a blood-curdling scream. If you have a stone, stick, or spray, that may be a helpful deterrent.

The most effective means of avoiding a vicious dog was related to us by marathoner Lou Castagnola.

"One day I was out on a long run on a narrow country road. The most vicious German shepherd I ever saw went after me. He must have thought I was juicy or something. Fortunately, a car approached. Flailing my arms, I stood in the middle of the dirt road and forced the car to stop. I hopped in and the motorist drove me to the next road."

glycogen from the muscles, the more glycogen the muscles can hold. Increased amounts of glycogen bound in the muscles increase endurance. A runner who has twice as much glycogen in his muscles before exercise may have twice as much endurance.

4. Run fast at least once a week

Fast running creates a shortage of oxygen, characterized by fast breathing and a rapid heart rate. This is called running anaerobically and also is good. To compensate for the oxygen shortfall, the body increases the blood supply by widening the blood vessels to increase the circulation to the heart. It is because of this process that heart attacks are rare in active athletes.

5. When you feel heavy-legged, don't run hard even if you've scheduled a hard day

If you attempt a workout your body cannot handle, an injury often results. A few years ago, I had a twenty-mile run scheduled on a day when my legs were still stiff and heavy from a workout two days earlier. Instead of taking the day off or running easily, I decided to run hard for three miles. Feeling somewhat guilty about the shortened distance, I pressed the pace. At two and a half miles, I heard a loud snap and felt a pain in my calf. I had pulled the tendon out of my calf muscle. It was six weeks before I could run hard again.

6. If you have localized pain that gets worse as you run, stop

Pain is nature's way of telling you that your body has had enough. If you ignore the pain, expect to be injured.

A former coach of the U.S. Olympic team believes his athletes should be hard-nosed and trains them that way. When an athlete complains that his leg hurts, the coach's usual retort is, "Run on the other leg." While his tough training methods helped many athletes achieve international recognition, his runners were frequently injured.

7. Stretch twice a day

If you stretch your muscles, you can run faster.

Every time you run hard, your muscles are mildly injured. With healing, the affected muscle shortens,

All Competitive Distance Runners Deplete

Two-time Olympic marathoner Ken Moore depletes his muscle glycogen with a thirty-mile run each Sunday.

During my racing career, my depletion runs were never over seventeen miles. It would take too long for me to recover from runs longer than that.
— GABE MIRKIN, M.D.

subjecting it to added tension. This increased tension makes the muscle more susceptible to injury, and stretching the muscle is a sure way to counteract it. All runners should stretch their hamstrings and their calves, the lower back and inner thighs. After you arise each morning, and before you run, you should perform each of the stretching exercises in Chapter 10 at least five times.

Since you're going to stretch before you run, you needn't waste extra time doing calisthenics to warm up. You can warm up by starting your run slowly and gradually increasing the pace. By starting slowly, you will gradually heat up your muscles, increase their blood supply, and make them more pliable and less susceptible to injury.

However, if you're in a race, you may not want to start slowly. Before the race, you should jog a few miles and gradually increase the pace as you run. Then you can start your race at full tilt.

The Running Program

After several weeks of jogging ten minutes a day, you are ready to begin training by running three times a week. Even though you will be training less often, it will take more effort. Before even thinking of running more than three days a week, concentrate on building up your hard days.

In the beginning, don't go out and try to run as fast as you can. You must first build up your endurance by performing plenty of slow background running. Running thickens the ligaments and tendons and makes them more resistant to injury.

Here is a sequence of running schedules to guide you. Each step is more demanding and will allow you to gauge your progress, even though you may not be competing against other runners.

Brett or Barbara the beginner

Sat.: Off
Sun.: Run 1 mile
Mon.: Off
Tues.: Run 1 mile
Wed.: Off
Thurs.: Run 1 mile
Fri.: Off
(Italics indicate hard days)

Stretching Is More Important Than Calisthenics

We don't do calisthenics. But since we started a refined stretching program two years ago, we haven't had a player miss a game due to a pulled leg muscle.

— GENE MONAHAN,
trainer for the 1977 world-champion New York Yankees

On your hard days, run fast enough to cause deep breathing. Do not try to run faster than that. Breathing too hard and fast will limit the number of miles you run.

Even though you are running less than you did in the pre-training program, you will be running at a faster pace. This will put more stress on your muscles and you must be very careful that you don't injure yourself.

Gradually add a half mile to your runs until your schedule looks like this:

Nick or Nora the novice

Sat.: Off
Sun.: Run 3 miles
Mon.: Off
Tues.: Run 2 miles
Wed.: Off
Thurs.: Run 2 miles
Fri.: Off

After a hard run you will feel good and sleep like a baby. The next morning your calves and hamstrings will feel tight. It is very important that you stretch these muscles. If you have the time, do it in the morning and always before you run.

After a few weeks of running only three times a week, you will want to run more. Start jogging on your easy days. Be careful not to run hard, because on these days you will be more susceptible to injury.

On easy days, don't set any specific distance or pace for yourself. And don't yield to the temptation of running fast. If you do, you may not be able to run hard on your next scheduled hard day.

You have now become:

Rupert or Rebecca the runner

Sat.: Jog
Sun.: Run 3 miles
Mon.: Jog
Tues.: Run 3 miles
Wed.: Jog
Thurs.: Run 2 miles
Fri.: Jog

Once you have established a daily program, your next goal is to build up mileage on your hard days. Your ultimate goal is to include a long, medium, and short run in your weekly program.

As your body dictates, gradually add a half mile to each hard day. Most runners run their long run on weekends. Everyone has his or her own rate of improvement. You will have many setbacks in your training and you must learn to listen to your body. Even though you may have had a seven-mile run last week, that distance may be too far for you this week.

If you are careful and listen to your body, your next goal is to become:

Carl or Carla the competitor

Sat.: Jog
Sun.: Run 10 miles
Mon.: Jog
Tues.: Run 3 miles
Wed.: Jog
Thurs.: Run 5 miles
Fri.: Jog

Notice that I do not recommend that you jog a specific distance on your easy days. If you feel good you can jog even up to ten miles. If your legs are stiff, you may jog only ten feet. Jog slowly and don't overdo it.

If you run just to feel good and to protect your health, you may not want to extend your training program any further. That will take more time and more effort. The next step is to race. To do so, join an organization. Almost every large city in the United States has a branch of the Road Runners Club.

For competition, a new training technique, called interval running, should be introduced. This involves running a fixed distance in a fixed time with a fixed recovery period. A good example: Running a quarter mile in 75 seconds with a 110-yard jog. Repeat ten times. This technique teaches the muscles to move faster and the speedometer in the brain adapts to faster running.

Many high school coaches use this technique — sometimes to excess. Only superbly conditioned athletes can run intervals more than once a week and still keep up their workload. The more fast intervals, the fewer miles you can run each week.

Many runners don't like the regimentation of a clock. They use a system called "fartlek" — a Swedish word

To Join the Road Runners Club

To find out the nearest branch of the Road Runners Club of America, send a stamped, self-addressed envelop to:

> Ellen Wessel, Director of
> Public Relations
> 1111 Army Navy Drive
> Arlington, Virginia 22202

Businesses for Fitness

Large businesses are budgeting money for running programs. They know that a heart attack to a key executive can cost the operation more than $750,000. It's obvious that it is cheaper to prevent disease than to treat it. That's why more than three hundred corporations in the United States have full-time directors of physical fitness.
— ED AYRES, *editor of*
Running Times *and co-author
of* The Bottom Line Benefit
of Corporate Fitness

meaning speed play. Using fartlek, you run fast when you feel like it; jog when you tire; and on recovering, run fast again. Fartlek combines numerous speed runs and slow jogs. Although fartlek is not as regimented as interval running, it requires a better knowledge of your body and a stronger will to promote maximum improvement. Fartlek is less likely to cause injury.

You are ready now for a schedule like this:

Ronald or Rachel the racer

Sat.: Jog 5 miles
Sun.: Run 10 miles
Mon.: Jog 5 miles
Tues.: Run 4 half-mile intervals with a quarter-mile jog between each; follow with a hard 6-mile run
Wed.: Jog 7 miles
Thurs.: Run 6 miles
Fri.: Jog 7 miles

Your program has progressed to fifty miles a week.

A serious high school distance runner will run between fifty and seventy miles a week. A good college competitor will cover more than seventy miles a week. International runners run more than one hundred miles a week.

At this level of training, your leg muscles will feel tight on the mornings after a hard day. But as the day goes on, your muscles will relax and feel stronger.

On the morning after an easy day, your body will be brimming with energy and you will actually hunger for each run. You will be surprised how important running has become to your life-style.

By the time you can run fifty or more miles per week, you are usually addicted to running. As soon as you lie down at night, you fall into a deep sleep. By going out for a long run, you can get rid of most of your problems for six to twenty-four hours. You will feel so good that missing even one day of running will cause you to feel jittery and nervous.

However, as occurs with most addictions, the magnificent high that you experience with each run can only be maintained by increasing the dosage. You will compulsively try to increase your mileage. However, your body can only tolerate so much work before it breaks down. At this point you must learn to listen to your body's warning signals or you will be injured most of the time.

By adding a four-mile jog on weekday mornings, you will progress up to seventy miles a week.

You should now be able to join many marathon runners with a schedule like this:

Marty or Martha the marathoner

Sat.: A.M., off. P.M., jog 5 miles
Sun.: A.M., run 12 miles. P.M., off
Mon.: A.M., jog 4 miles. P.M., jog 5 miles
Tues.: A.M., jog 4 miles. P.M., run 4 half-mile intervals with quarter-mile jogs in between followed by a hard 6-mile run
Wed.: A.M., jog 4 miles. P.M., jog 7 miles
Thurs.: A.M., jog 4 miles. P.M., run 6 miles
Fri.: A.M., jog 4 miles. P.M., jog 7 miles
Total = 70+ miles a week.

Too much mileage can be harmful. Bodies break down on mileage between 150 and 200 miles a week. I know of no international competitors who are able to continue running more than 150 miles a week over many years.

America's Love Affair with the Marathon

YEAR	NUMBER OF MARATHONS	ENTRANTS	ENTRANTS RUNNING MARATHON IN LESS THAN 3 HOURS
1966	12	1,500	150
1970	73	8,000	812
1977	197	25,000	4,000
1978	320	60,000	6,000

There is almost one marathon per day in the United States this year.

Source: Figures courtesy of *Running Times*.

If you can match this training schedule, you will become a successful marathon runner. We'll call you:

Elwood or Ellen the elite

Sat.: A.M., off. P.M., jog 10 miles
Sun.: A.M., run 30 miles. P.M., off
Mon.: A.M., jog 5 miles. P.M., jog 7 miles

Tues.: A.M., jog 5 miles. P.M., run 4 half-mile intervals with quarter-mile jogs in between; follow with a hard 7-mile run

Wed.: A.M., jog 5 miles. P.M., jog 7 miles

Thurs.: A.M., jog 5 miles. P.M., run 10 miles

Fri.: A.M., jog 5 miles. P.M., jog 7 miles

This schedule adds up to 106 miles per week. On a continued basis, I was never able to run more than 100 miles a week. If you can run these workouts, you don't need any further advice from me. You will run farther and faster than I ever did.

Appendix A
Members of the American Orthopaedic Society for Sports Medicine

ALABAMA

John B. Morris, M.D.
7833 Second Avenue South
Birmingham, Alabama 35206

Ernest C. Brock, M.D.
535 River Road East
Tuscaloosa, Alabama 35401

R. Joe Burleson, M.D.
Box 6291, CCHS,
University of Alabama
University, Alabama 35486

ARIZONA

Tom P. Coker, M.D.
P.O. Drawer 1608, 2907 East Joyce
Fayetteville, Arizona 72701

H. Austin Grimes, M.D.
12th & Van Buren Streets
Little Rock, Arizona 72205

Kenneth G. Jones, M.D.
P.O. Box 5270
12th & Van Buren Streets
Little Rock, Arizona 72205

James G. Garrick, M.D.
333 East Virginia Avenue, #101
Phoenix, Arizona 85004

George F. Hewson, Jr., M.D.
2102 Country Club Road
Tucson, Arizona 85716

Edward C. Percy, M.D.
Arizona Health Science Center
Tucson, Arizona 85724

CALIFORNIA

Phillip H. McFarland, M.D.
101 Laguna Road
Fullerton, California 92635

Vincent S. Carter, M.D.
575 East Hardy Street
Inglewood, California 90301

H. Royer Collins, M.D.
575 East Hardy Street
Inglewood, California 90301

Anthony F. Daly, M.D.
233 North Prairie Avenue
Inglewood, California 90301

Frank W. Jobe, M.D.
575 East Hardy Street
Inglewood, California 90301

Robert Kerlan, M.D.
575 East Hardy Street
Inglewood, California 90301

Clarence L. Shields, Jr., M.D.
575 East Hardy Street
Inglewood, California 90301

Theodore R. Waugh, M.D.
University of California
Department of Surgery
Irvine, California 92664

Douglas W. Jackson, M.D.
2840 Long Beach Boulevard, #410
Long Beach, California 90806

J. Mayfield Harris, M.D.
793 Altos Oaks Drive
Los Altos, California 94022

Sonny P. Cobble, M.D.
2300 South Hope Street, Suite 100
Los Angeles, California 90007

Gerald A. M. Finerman, M.D.
University of California
Center for Health Sciences
Los Angeles, California 90024

J. Harold LaBriola, M.D.
8540 Sepulveda
Los Angeles, California 90045

Sanford H. Anzel, M.D.
1201 West La Veta Avenue
Orange, California 92668

Fred L. Behling, M.D.
300 Homer Avenue
Palo Alto, California 94301

John J. O'Hara, M.D.
923 South Catalina Avenue
Redondo Beach, California 90277

H. Paul Bauer, Jr., M.D.
Midway Medical Center
3405 Kenyon Street, Suite 405
Sandiego, California 92110

Robert W. Straumfjord, M.D.
2850 Sixth Avenue
San Diego, California 92103

E. Paul Woodward, M.D.
7920 Frost Street
San Diego, California 92123

Michael W. Chapman, M.D.
1001 Potrero Avenue
San Francisco, California 94110

James M. Glick, M.D.
2299 Post Street
San Francisco, California 94115

John H. Nadeau, M.D.
160 Country Club Drive
South San Francisco
California 94080

Grady L. Jeter, M.D.
2430 Samaritan Drive
San Jose, California 95124

Martin Trieb, M.D.
2430 Samaritan Drive
San Jose, California 95124

Robert S. Watanabe, M.D.
2901 Wilshire Boulevard, #221
Santa Monica, California 90403

Martin E. Blazina, M.D.
4911 Van Nuys Boulevard, #104
Sherman Oaks, California 91403

J. R. Steadman, M.D.
P.O. Box 10708
South Lake Tahoe, California 95731

Edward M. Tapper, M.D.
P.O. Box 10708
South Lake Tahoe, California 95731

R. T. Nussdorf, M.D.
12522 East Lambert Road
Whittier, California 90606

COLORADO

Robert R. Oden, M.D.
100 East Main Street
P.O. Box 660
Aspen Colorado 81611

Charles W. Brown, M.D.
1830 Williams Street
Denver, Colorado 80218

John D. Leidholt, M.D.
2045 Franklin Street
Denver Colorado 80205

Robert P. Mack, M.D.
2045 Franklin Street
Denver, Colorado 80205

Richard Talbott, M.D.
1707 East 18th Street
Denver, Colorado 80218

Courtney W. Brown, M.D.
1785 Kipling Street
Lakewood, Colorado 80215

Duane G. Messner, M.D.
1785 Kipling Street
Lakewood, Colorado 80215

CONNECTICUT

William A. Sinton, M.D.
85 Osborn Street
Danbury, Connecticut 06810

Gary A. Gallo, M.D.
20 Dayton Avenue
Greenwich, Connecticut 06830

James F. Donovan, M.D.
85 Jefferson Street
Hartford, Connecticut 06106

Vincent J. Turco, M.D.
140 Woodland Street
Hartford, Connecticut 06105

William J. Waskowitz, M.D.
40 Hart Street
New Britain, Connecticut 06052

Norman A. Zlotzky, M.D.
23 Elm Street
Rockville, Connecticut 06066

DISTRICT OF COLUMBIA

Major P. Gladden, M.D.
2018 Georgia Avenue, N.W.
Washington, D.C. 20001

Stanford A. Lavine, M.D.
1145-19th Street, N.W., #300
Washington, D.C. 20036

FLORIDA

Phillip L. Parr, M.D.
923 N.W. 13th Street
Gainesville, Florida 32601

Jaime M. Benavides, M.D.
P.O. Box 1240
Key West, Florida 33040

Arthur J. Pearl, M.D.
9106 S.W. 87th Avenue
Miami, Florida 33156

Hugh S. Unger, M.D.
16501 N.W. Second Avenue
North Miami Beach, Florida 33169

Paul F. Wallace, M.D.
1501 Fifth Avenue, North
Saint Petersburg, Florida 33705

Harold L. Williamson, M.D.
602 South Howard Avenue
Tampa, Florida 33606

Donald L. Ames, M.D.
736-22nd Place
Vero Beach, Florida 32960

George L. Ford, Jr., M.D.
5312 Broadway
West Palm Beach, Florida 33407

Richard D. Hoover, M.D.
5312 Broadway
West Palm Beach, Florida 33407

GEORGIA

William B. Mulherin, M.D.
125 King Avenue
Athens, Georgia 30601

Fred L. Allman, Jr., M.D.
615 Peachtree Street
Atlanta, Georgia 30308

F. James Funk, Jr., M.D.
1938 Peachtree Road, N.W.
Atlanta, Georgia 30309

Robert E. Wells, M.D.
1938 Peachtree Road, N.W.
Atlanta, Georgia 30309

Robert L. Brand, M.D.
1132 Druid Park Avenue
Augusta, Georgia 30904

Hamlin Graham, M.D.
1021 15th Street
Augusta, Georgia 30901

James R. Andrews, M.D.
105 Physicians Building
Columbus, Georgia 31901

Jack C. Hughston, M.D.
105 Physicians Building
Columbus, Georgia 31901

IDAHO

Gilbert A. Bacon, M.D.
352 East Center Street
Pocatello, Idaho 83201

ILLINOIS

David C. Bachman, M.D.
233 East Erie Street, #700
Chicago, Illinois 60611

Clint Compere, M.D.
233 East Erie Street
Chicago, Illinois 60611

Bernard R. Cahill, M.D.
416 St. Mark Court
Peoria, Illinois 61603

INDIANA

Bryant A. Bloss, M.D.
801 St. Mary's Drive
Evansville, Indiana 47715

Thomas A. Brady, M.D.
1815 North Capitol Avenue
Indianapolis, Indiana 46202

George F. Rapp, M.D.
8402 Harcourt Road
Suite 809
Indianapolis, Indiana 46260

William B. Ferguson, M.D.
2525 South Street
Lafayette Orthopaedic Clinic
Lafayette, Indiana 47904

Alois E. Gibson, M.D.
1250 Chester Boulevard
Richmond, Indiana 47374

Leslie M. Bodnar, M.D.
328 North Michigan Street
South Bend, Indiana 46601

Albert F. Dingley, Jr., M.D.
109 South St. Louis Avenue
South Bend, Indiana 46617

IOWA

John P. Albright, M.D.
C106 Children's Hospital
University of Iowa Hospital
Iowa City, Iowa 52242

KANSAS

Charles E. Henning, M.D.
320 North Hillside
Witchita, Kansas 67214

KENTUCKY

D. Kay Clawson, M.D.
University of Kentucky
College of Medicine, MN140
Lexington, Kentucky 40506

William G. Wheeler, M.D.
2537 Larkin Road
Lexington, Kentucky 40503

Rudy J. Ellis, M.D.
Medical Towers South, #364
234 East Gray Street
Louisville, Kentucky 40202

LOUISIANA

Alvin Stander, M.D.
5630 Bankers Avenue
Baton Rouge, Louisiana 70808

David, J. Drez, Jr., M.D.
2800 Second Avenue
Lake Charles, Louisiana 70601

Robert D. D'Ambrosia, M.D.
1524 Tulane Avenue
New Orleans, Louisiana 70112

Ray J. Haddad, Jr., M.D.
2633 Napolean Avenue
New Orleans, Louisiana 70115

J. Kenneth Saer, M.D.
1538 Louisiana Avenue
New Orleans, Louisiana 70115

William S. Bundrick, M.D.
835 Margaret Place
Shreveport, 71101

MAINE

Lawrence Crane, M.D.
157 Pine Street
Portland, Maine 04102

MARYLAND

Jay Shelton Cox, M.D.
Captain MC USN Naval Hospital
Annapolis, Maryland 21402

Edmond J. McDonnell, M.D.
4 East Madison Street
Baltimore, Maryland 21202

Charles E. Silberstein, M.D.
4 East Madison Street
Baltimore, Maryland 21202

Robert R. R. Roberts, M.D.
801 Toll House Avenue
Frederick, Maryland 21701

Wayne B. Leadbetter, M.D.
8830 Cameron Street
Silver Spring, Maryland 20910

The Sportsmedicine Institute
9900 Georgia Avenue
Silver Spring, Maryland 20902
(301) 589-0599

MASSACHUSETTS

Joseph R. Rokous, M.D.
140 Haverhill Street
Andover, Massachusetts 01810

Robert E. Leach, M.D.
750 Harrison Avenue
Boston, Massachusetts 02118

Dinesh Patel, M.D.
266 Beacon Street
Boston, Massachusetts 02116

Donald S. Pierce, M.D.
275 Charles Street
Boston, Massachusetts 02114

Carter R. Rowe, M.D.
275 Charles Street
Boston, Massachusetts 02114

John F. Duff, M.D.
4 State Road
Danvers, Massachusetts 01923

George Snook, M.D.
264 Elm Street
Northampton, Massachusetts 01060

Arthur E. Ellison, M.D.
Adams Road
Williamstown, Massachusetts 01267

MICHIGAN

Robert Bailey, M.D.
University Hospital
Room C4127
Ann Arbor, Michigan 48104

Gerald A. O'Connor, M.D.
P.O. Box 994
Ann Arbor, Michigan 48106

Thomas R. Peterson, M.D.
2015 Manchester Road
Ann Arbor, Michigan 48104

Edwin R. Guise, Jr., M.D.
Henry Ford Hospital
2799 West Grand Boulevard
Detroit, Michigan 48202

Melvin D. Wolf, M.D.
G-3083 Flushing Road
Flint, Michigan 48504

Perry W. Greene, Jr., M.D.
1900 Wealthy Street, S.E.
Grand Rapids, Michigan 49506

Robert C. Mahaney, M.D.
714 Michigan Avenue
Holland, Michigan 49423

Ben R. Mayne, M.D.
2111 Marshall Court
Saginaw, Michigan 48602

Waldomar Roesser, M.D.
5305 East Huron River Drive
Suite 3-B100
Ypsilanti, Michigan 48192

MINNESOTA

E. Harvey O'Phelan, M.D.
825 South Eighth Street
Minneapolis, Minnesota 55404

Franklin H. Sim, M.D.
200 First Street, S.W.
Rochester, Minnesota 55901

MISSISSIPPI

Wiley C. Hutchins, M.D.
P.O. Box 721
Columbus, Mississippi 39701

William C. Warner, M.D.
727 Carlisle Street
Jackson, Mississippi 39202

Wayne T. Lamar, M.D.
2168 South Lamar
Oxford, Mississippi 38655

MISSOURI

William C. Allen, M.D.
University of Missouri
Medical Center N-502
Columbia, Missouri 65201

Dale E. Darnell, M.D.
4320 Wornall Road
Kansas City, Missouri 64111

Gael R. Frank, M.D.
4240 Blue Ridge Boulevard
501 Blue Ridge Tower
Kansas City, Missouri 64133

Paul W. Meyer, M.D.
4320 Wornall Road
Kansas City, Missouri 64111

NEBRASKA

John G. Yost, M.D.
606 North Minnesota
Hastings, Nebraska 68901

NEVADA

Gerald L. Dales, Jr., M.D.
633 North Arlington Avenue
Reno, Nevada 89503

NEW HAMPSHIRE

Robert E. Porter, M.D.
2 Maynard Street
Hanover, New Hampshire 03755

NEW JERSEY

Cornelius N. Stover, M.D.
Hunterdon Medical Center
Flemington, New Jersey 08822

Joseph J. O'Conner, M.D.
285 Henry Street
Orange, New Jersey 07050

Max Novich, M.D.
313 State Street
Perth Amboy, New Jersey 08861

Raymond L. Cunneff, M.D.
21 East Front Street
Red Bank, New Jersey 07701

NEW MEXICO

John F. Boyd, M.D.
1025 Medical Arts Street, N.E.
Albuquerque, New Mexico 87102

Barry R. Maron, M.D.
4221 Silver Avenue, S.E.
Albuquerque, New Mexico 87108

NEW YORK

Arthur M. Bernhang, M.D.
124 Main Street
Huntington, New York 11743

Burton L. Berson, M.D.
1100 Park Avenue
New York, New York 10028

J. William Fielding, M.D.
105 East 65th Street
New York, New York 10021

William G. Hamilton, M.D.
345 West 58th Street
New York, New York 10019

William Liebler, M.D.
742 Park Avenue
New York, New York 10021

John L. Marshall, M.D.
535 East 70th Street
New York, New York 10021

Jeffrey Minkoff, M.D.
130 East 77th Street
New York, New York 10021

James A. Nicholas, M.D.
130 East 77th Street
New York, New York 10021

Russell F. Warren, M.D.
535 East 70th Street
New York, New York 10021

Joseph D. Godfrey, M.D.
South 3669 Southwestern Boulevard
Orchard Park, New York 14127

Richard L. Weiss, M.D.
South 3669 Southwestern Boulevard
Orchard Park, New York 14127

Kenneth E. DeHaven, M.D.
601 Elmwood Avenue
Rochester, New York 14642

Jerome L. Meisel, M.D.
Kohl Professional Building
Route 59
Suffern, New York 10901

Bruce E. Baker, M.D.
750 East Adams Street
Syracuse, New York 13201

John A. Feagin, Jr., M.D.
Qtrs. 76-A Schofield Place
West Point, New York 10996

Robert R. Protzman, M.D.
U. S. Military Academy
West Point, New York 10996

NORTH CAROLINA

Wayne S. Montgomery, M.D.
Doctors Drive
Asheville, North Carolina 28801

Basil M. Boyd, Jr., M.D.
1822 Brunswick Avenue
Charlotte, North Carolina 28207

David S. Johnston, M.D.
1822 Brunswick Avenue
Charlotte, North Carolina 28207

F. Wayne Lee, M.D.
225 Hawthorne Lane
Charlotte, North Carolina 28204

Angus McBride, Jr., M.D.
1822 Brunswick Avenue
Charlotte, North Carolina 28207

Frank H. Bassett, III, M.D.
Duke Hospital–West Unit
3100 Eribin Road
Durham, North Carolina 27710

James F. Bowman, M.D.
210 West Fourth Street
Greenville, North Carolina 27834

Stephen H. Homer, M.D.
3111 Maplewood Avenue, #104
Winston-Salem, North Carolina
27103

George D. Rovere, M.D.
Bowman Gray School of Medicine
Winston-Salem, North Carolina
27103

OHIO

George J. Mallo, M.D.
640 West Market Street
Akron, Ohio 44303

E. Herbert Thompson, M.D.
640 West Market Street
Akron, Ohio 44303

Frank R. Noyes, M.D.
Room 346 Medical Sciences Building
231 Bethesda Avenue
Cincinnati, Ohio 45267

John A. Bergfeld, M.D.
9500 Euclid Avenue
Cleveland, Ohio 44106

Malcolm Brahms, M.D.
11811 Shaker Boulevard
Cleveland, Ohio 44120

John E. Leach, M.D.
1275 Olentangy River Road
Columbus, Ohio 43212

Mel L. Olix, M.D.
3600 Olentangy River Road
Columbus, Ohio 43214

Richard F. Slager, M.D.
1300 Dublin Road
Columbus, Ohio 43215

David M. Bell, M.D.
14701 Detroit Avenue
Lakewood, Ohio 44107

Gerald W. Sutherland, M.D.
4747 Holland-Sylvania Road
Sylvania, Ohio 43560

OKLAHOMA

James P. Bell, M.D.
600 N.W. 11th Street
Oklahoma City, Oklahoma 73106

Don H. O'Donoghue, M.D.
217 Pasteur Medical Building
Oklahoma City, Oklahoma 73103

George S. Mauerman, M.D.
6565 South Yale Avenue, #1212
Tulsa, Oklahoma 74136

James E. White, M.D.
6565 South Yale Avenue
Tulsa, Oklahoma 74136

OREGON

Stanley L. James, M.D.
750 East 11th Avenue
Eugene, Oregon 97401

Robert L. Larson
750 East 11th Avenue
Eugene, Oregon 97401

Donald Slocum, M.D.
750 East 11th Avenue
Eugene, Oregon 97401

Charles A. Fagan, M.D.
9155 S.W. Barnes Road, #202
Portland, Oregon 97225

Thomas E. Fagan, M.D.
5415 S.W. Westgate Drive
Portland, Oregon 97221

Thad C. Stanford, M.D.
873 Medical Center Drive
Salem, Oregon 97301

PENNSYLVANIA

Alexander Kalenak, M.D.
Hershey Medical Center
Hershey, Pennsylvania 17033

Vincent J. DiStefano, M.D.
419 South 19th Street
Philadelphia, Pennsylvania 19146

James Nixon, M.D.
415 South 19th Street
Philadelphia, Pennsylvania 19146

Joseph S. Torg, M.D.
3401 North Broad Street
Philadelphia, Pennsylvania 19140

James H. McMaster, M.D.
Allegheny General Hospital
320 East North Avenue
Pittsburgh, Pennsylvania 15212

Charles S. Stone, M.D.
128 North Craig Street
Pittsburgh, Pennsylvania 15213

Richard W. Godshall, M.D.
Lawn Avenue Professional Building
Box 192
Sellersville, Pennsylvania 18960

RHODE ISLAND

Americo Savastano, M.D.
205 Waterman Street
Providence, Rhode Island 02906

SOUTH CAROLINA

William B. Evins, Jr., M.D.
101 Chapman Street
Greenville, South Carolina 29605

Roland Knight, M.D.
101 Chapman Street
Greenville, South Carolina 29605

TENNESSEE

Robert C. Coddington, M.D.
Doctors Building, Suite 317
Chattanooga, Tennessee 37402

Walter C. Chapman, M.D.
223 North Main Street
Greeneville, Tennessee 37743

Howell H. Sherrod, M.D.
202 West Watauga
Johnson City, Tennessee 37601

Robert Brashear, M.D.
P.O. Box 11047
630 Concord Street, S.W.
Knoxville, Tennessee 37919

Roy A. Wedekind, M.D.
8813 Wessex Drive
Knoxville, Tennessee 37919

Williams Youmans, M.D.
630 Concord Street, S.W.
Knoxville, Tennessee 37919

Robert H. Haralson, III, M.D.
822 Tuckaleechee Pike
Maryville, Tennessee 37801

Phillip M. Aronoff, M.D.
969 Madison Avenue, #1403
Memphis, Tennessee 38104

T. David Sisk, M.D.
869 Madison Avenue
Memphis, Tennessee 38104

Marcus J. Stewart, M.D.
869 Madison Avenue
Memphis, Tennessee 38104

A. Brant Lipscomb, M.D.
St. Thomas Medical Building, #213
4230 Harding Road
Nashville, Tennessee 37205

Elwood J. Eichler, M.D.
1011 East 32nd Street
Austin, Texas 78705

Jerry D. Julian, M.D.
3100 Red River
Austin, Texas 78705

James W. Shuffield, M.D.
3650 Laurel
Beaumont, Texas 77707

Stonie R. Cotten, M.D.
2601 Welborn Street
Dallas, Texas 75219

James P. Evans, M.D.
9262 Forest Lane
Dallas, Texas 75231

John B. Gunn, M.D.
3600 Gaston Avenue, #303
Dallas, Texas 75246

Gerald W. Schofield, M.D.
1000 Emerald Isle, #110
Dallas, Texas 75218

Harold J. Brelsford, M.D.
2210 Maroneal
Houston, Texas 77030

James E. Butler, M.D.
6410 Fannin Street
Houston, Texas 77030

Thomas E. Cain, M.D.
2210 Maroneal
Houston, Texas 77030

A. Ross Davis, M.D.
1213 Hermann Drive, #470
Houston, Texas 77004

Robert H. Fain, M.D.
2210 Maroneal
Houston, Texas 77030

Joe W. King, M.D.
7719 Buffalo Speedway
Houston, Texas 77025

Edward T. Smith, M.D.
2120 Brentwood
Houston, Texas 77030

Jack Southern, M.D.
2210 Maroneal
Houston, Texas 77030

Rufus F. Stanley, M.D.
6535 Fannin Street
Houston, Texas 77030

Hugh Tullos, M.D.
6535 Fannin Street
Houston, Texas 77030

Emmet Shannon, M.D.
3801-19th Street
Lubbock, Texas 79410

Lamar P. Collie, M.D.
1303 McCullough
San Antonio, Texas 78212

Jack Hopkins Henry, M.D.
8038 Wurzbach Road
San Antonio, Texas 78229

John Hinchey, M.D.
1303 McCullough
San Antonio, Texas 78212

Charles A. Rockwood, Jr., M.D.
University of Texas
Medical School
San Antonio, Texas 78284

Ray W. Covington, M.D.
3500 Hillcrest Drive
Waco, Texas 76708

John R. Merendino, M.D.
Moreau Medical Building
1002 East South Temple
Salt Lake City, Utah 84102

Robert J. Johnson, M.D.
University of Vermont
Medical School
Burlington, Vermont 05401

John T. Hulvey, M.D.
211 West Main Street
Abington, Virginia 24210

Robert P. Nirschl, M.D.
3801 North Fairfax Drive
Arlington, Virginia 22203

Frank C. McCue, III, M.D.
Department of Orthopedics and Reha-
   bilitation
Box 243, University of Virginia
   Medical Center
Charlottesville, Virginia 22901

Gervas S. Taylor, Jr., M.D.
844 Kempsville Road, Suite 101
Norfolk, Virginia 23502

E. L. Clements, Jr., M.D.
4315 Grove Avenue
Richmond, Virginia 23221

Virgil R. May, Jr., M.D.
2222 Monument Avenue
Richmond, Virginia 23220

George P. Ripley, M.D.
1240 Third Street, S.W.
Roanoke, Virginia 24016

P. M. Palumbo, M.D.
8206 Leesburg Pike
Tyson Corner, Virginia 22180

Victor H. Frankel, M.D.
Department of Orthopaedics–RK-1C
University of Washington
Seattle, Washington 98195

Harry H. Kretzler, Jr., M.D.
1207-200th Street
Seattle, Washington 98133

Stanley A. Mueller, Jr., M.D.
212 South J Street
Tacoma, Washington 98405

K. Douglas Bowers, Jr., M.D.
400 Drummond Street
Morgantown, West Virginia 26505

WISCONSIN

William G. Clancy, Jr., M.D.
1300 University Avenue
Madison, Wisconsin 53706

Bruce J. Brewer, M.D.
8700 West Wisconsin Avenue
Milwaukee, Wisconsin 53226

Gary N. Guten, M.D.
1218 West Kilbourn Avenue
Milwaukee, Wisconsin 53233

CANADA

Peter John Fowler, M.D.
111 Waterloo Street
London 15, Ontario

Jack C. Kennedy, M.D.
111 Waterloo Street
London 15, Ontario

Carroll A. Laurin, M.D.
3875 Rue St., Urbain 109
Montreal 131, Quebec

James E. Bateman, M.D.
40 Wellesley Street East
Toronto 5, Ontario

Source: American Orthopaedic Society for Sports Medicine, 430 North Michigan Ave., Chicago, Illinois 60611. Reprinted by permission.

Appendix B
American Academy of Podiatric Sports Medicine Membership List

Unless otherwise stated, all physicians listed here are D.P.M.s.

ALABAMA

William A. Wood
1045 Forrest Avenue
Gadsdan, Alabama 35901
(205) 822-7220

David J. Landau
Todd Shopping Mall
Suite 2025
Vestavia Hills, Alabama 35216
(205) 822-7220

ARIZONA

Alexander T. Borgeas
129 West Catalina Drive
Phoenix, Arizona 85013
(602) 264-4100

M. R. Davidson
1028 East McDowell Road
Phoenix, Arizona 85066
(602) 252-1110

Gerald L. Campbell
2210 South Mill Avenue, #7
Tempe, Arizona 85282
(602) 968-7707

Jonathan M. Singer
600 West 16th Street
Yuma, Arizona 85364

CALIFORNIA

Michael J. Schnitzer
1120 West La Palma Avenue
Suite 12
Anaheim, California 92801
(714) 991-6770

R. Bruce Franz
509 West 18th Street
Antioch, California 94509
(415) 737-1028

Robert N. Mohr
435 North Bedford Drive, #102
Beverly Hills, California 90210
(213) 273-0532

ROBERT M. BARNES*
1130 West Olive Avenue
Burbank, California 91506
(213) 848-1202

FRANCIS A. LANTZ*
3039 Jefferson
Carlsbad, California 92008

Brian A. McDowell
6401 Coyle Avenue
Carmichael, California 95608

Ben Hara
1257 West San Bernardino Road
Covina, California 91722
(213) 331-7391

Franklin Kase
6400 Green Valley Circle, #2-304
Culver City, California 90230

John M. Connolly
48 Park Plaza Drive
Suite 301
Daly City, California 94015
(415) 756-1631

Federico R. Hernandez
509 South Eighth Street
El Centro, California 92243
(714) 352-6062

Frank W. Swierupski
23321 El Roro Road
Suite C
El Toro, California 92630

Warren M. Johnson
3200 Mowry Avenue
Suite B
Fremont, California 94538
(415) 794-6633

Martin E. Serbin
1001 South Brookhurst Road
Fullerton, California 92633

Robert Basinger
27171 Calaroga Avenue, #4
Hayward, California 94545

William E. Stahl
1419 B Street
Hayward, California 94541
(415) 581-1601

STEVEN I. SUBOTNICK*
19682 Hesperian Boulevard
Hayward, California 94541
(415) 783-3255

John P. Jesse
662 25th Street
Hermosa Beach, California 90254

Dennis R. Gumm
4181 Branford Drive
Huntington Beach, California 92649
(714) 846-8589

Joesph Ellis
7720 Herschel
La Jolla, California 92037

PAUL CALIFANO*
7170 University Avenue
La Mesa, California 92041

Burr McKeehan
23561 Paseo de Valencia, #21
Laguna Hills, California 92653

Kenneth M. Teshima
23561 Paseo de Valencia, #21
Laguna Hills, California
(714) 837-2121

THOMAS AMBERRY*
2454 Atlantic Avenue
Long Beach, California 90806

Richard L. Bell
203 Covina Avenue
Long Beach, California 90803
(213) 434-8715

JOHN W. PAGLIANO*
4301 Atlantic Avenue
Suite 6
Long Beach, California 90807
(213) 426-0376

Michael S. Blair
1001 Gayley Avenue
Suite 105
Los Angeles, CA 90024
(213) 479-3226

ROBERT L. BRENNAN*
4201 Wilshire Boulevard
Los Angeles, California 90010

Charles R. Brantingham
3791 Katella, #207
Los Alamites, California 90720
(213) 430-1084

William G. Gerlach
202 Britton Way
Mather Air Force Base,
  California 95655

James F. Dietz
36 Tiburon Boulevard
Mill Valley, California 94941
(415) 388-0650

HARRY F. HLAVAC*
36 Tiburon Boulevard
Mill Valley, California 94941
(415) 388-0650

Richard Schiller
36 Tiburon Boulevard
Mill Valley, California 94941
(415) 388-0650

Craig E. Lowe
355 Placetia Avenue
Suite 105
Newport Beach, California 92663

Arthur A. Walton
745 Dover Drive, #4
Newport Beach, California 92663
(714) 548-5121

Russel J. Wojcik
5624 Gentry
North Hollywood, California 91607

Wesley J. Endo
2832 Summit Street
Oakland, California 94609

Mark A. Wolpa
400 40th Street
Oakland, California 94609

Michael Small
735 North A Street
Oxnard, California 93030

Charles H. Johnson
4009 Brockton Avenue
Riverside, California 92504
(714) 686-6798

Mitchell Mosher
120 Ascot Drive
Roseville, California 95678

Randall J. Sarte
2322 Butano Drive
Suite 224
Sacramento, California 95821

Douglas H. Freer
1855 Evergreen Street
San Diego, California 92106

RICHARD S. GILBERT*
3363 4th Avenue
San Diego, California 92103
(714) 299-2870

Maurice J. Papier
4944 B Newport Avenue
San Diego, California 92107

JEROME A. WISNIEW*
625 Broadway Street, #406
San Diego, California 92101

Gerald Strange
45 Castro Street, #232
San Francisco, California 94114

Dennis F. Augustine
1231 Park Avenue
San Jose, California 95126

THOMAS SGARLATO*
100 O'Connor Drive, #2
San Jose, California 95128
(408) 275-1805

Tilden Sokoloff
433 Estudillo, #104
San Leandro, California 94577

Barry Rodgveller
1300 West Sixth Street
San Pedro, California 90732

Nathan Stein
1300 West Sixth Street
San Pedro, California 90732
(414) 831-0728

Chris Tintocolis
1919 State Street
Suite 105
Santa Barbara, California 93101

Jens Birkholm
801 East Chapel Street, #6
Santa Maria, California 93454

Daniel L. Altchuler
1243 Seventh Street
Santa Monica, California 90402

Richard T. Koenigsberg
500 East Remington Drive
Suite 18
Sunnyvale, California 94087

HOWARD J. MARSHALL*
6900 Foothill Boulevard
Tujunga, California 91042

Glenn A. Ocker
1148 San Bernardino Road
Upland, California 91786
(714) 985-1831

COLORADO

Victor M. Peterson
11000 East Yale Avenue
Aurora, Colorado 80014
(303) 751-7822

Barry A. Mittelman
P.O. Box 93
United States
  Air Force Academy, Colorado
  80840
(303) 472-5040

Gerald R. Travers
720 Tejon
Colorado Springs, Colorado 80902
(303) 475-8080

David F. Holz
7090 East Hampden
Denver, Colorado 80224
(303) 758-9031

David Wolf
7090 East Hampden
Denver, Colorado 80224
(303) 758-9031

CONNECTICUT

JEFFREY YALE*
364 East Main Street
Ansonia, Connecticut 06401
(203) 734-4806

Kenneth R. Kierstein
182 Montauk Avenue
New London, Connecticut 06320
(203) 447-1488

ROBERT F. WEISS*
Colony Street
Norwalk, Connecticut 06851
(203) 866-3377

ROBERT R. RINALDI*
24 Third Street
Stamford, Connecticut 06905
(203) 323-1171

MICHAEL SABIA, JR.*
24 Third Street
Stamford, Connecticut 06905
(203) 323-1171

Daniel C. Dobas
11 London Terrace
Stratford, Connecticut 06497

Steven R. Colsen
P.O. Box 275
Waterford, Connecticut 06385
(203) 443-2833

Irwin Kove
309 North Main Street
West Hartford, Connecticut 06117
(203) 233-7225

DISTRICT OF COLUMBIA

Harold B. Glickman
1145 19th Street, N.W.
Suite 508
Washington, D.C. 20036

George C. Ibars
2153 California Street, N.W.
Washington, D.C. 20008

Stanley R. Spund
4325 49th Street, N.W.
Washington, D.C. 20016
(202) 362-2883

FLORIDA

David Cantor
475 Biltmore Way
Suite 205
Coral Gables, Florida 33134

Steven L. Kringold
475 Biltmore Way
Suite 205
Coral Gables, Florida 33134

Michael Hornstein
928 D. Mar-West Drive
Fort Walton Beach, Florida 32548

ROBERT A. GIUDICE*
118 Southwest Fourth Avenue
Gainsville, Florida 32601

Joel F. Katz
4001 Newberry Road
Building D
Suite 111
Gainsville, Florida 32607
(904) 373-3077

Arthur B. Korbel
1959 South Ocean Drive
Hallandale, Florida 33009
(305) 458-5155

Harvey A. Pearl
3809 University Boulevard West
Jacksonville, Florida 32217
(904) 737-4166

Jared P. Frankel
3500 North State Road
Suite 7
Lauderdale Lakes, Florida 33319

JOSEPH DOLLAR*
211 East New Haven Avenue
Melbourne, Florida 32901
(305) 723-2022

JERALD FISHBEIN*
1040 71st Street
Miami, Florida 33141

Robert I. Gamet
6201 S.W. 70th Street
Miami, Florida 33143
(305) 667-5683

Keith B. Kashuk
6201 S.W. 70th Street
Miami, Florida 33143
(305) 667-5683

James R. Lindsey
4852 N.W. 7th Avenue
Miami, Florida 33127
(305) 751-9631

GORDON W. FALKNOR*
642 North Beach
Ormond Beach, Florida 32074

Irwin I. Ayes
6536 Central Avenue
St. Petersburg, Florida 33707
(813) 384-1551

David H. Gross
5622 Central Avenue
St. Petersburg, Florida 33707
(813) 345-0183

Larry J. Kipp
211 Bullard Parkway
Temple Terrace, Florida 33617
(813) 988-4801

Michael H. Katz
31 Nokomis Avenue South
Suite 103
Venice, Florida 33595
(813) 484-2602

GEORGIA

Irving H. Miller
401 Peachtree Street, N.W.
Suite 404
Atlanta, Georgia 30308

Richard L. Freeman
P.O. Box 80721
Chamblee, Georgia 30366

William F. Faddock
2982 Church Street
Suite 104
East Point, Georgia 30344

Michael J. Solomon
1300 Plaza Drive, #12
Lawrence, Georgia 30245
(409) 963-1802

Thomas S. Union
1101 River North Boulevard
Macon, Georgia 31211
(912) 742-3631

Alan H. Shaw
2550 Windy Hill Road, #202
Marietta, Georgia 30067
(404) 952-2040

Dalton McGlamry
1649 Brocheet Road
Tucker, Georgia 30084

Samuel R. Miller
697 Reading Avenue
West Reading, Georgia 19611
(215) 373-4154

HAWAII

Donald A. Guimont
35 Kainehe Street
Kailua, Oahu, Hawaii 96734
(808) 261-9931

ILLINOIS

Leonard Winston
6426 North Western
Chicago, Illinois 64645
(312) 274-1878

ROBERT A. BIEL*
800 Halstead Street
Chicago Heights, Illinois 60411

Stephen Smith
420 Lee Street
Des Plaines, Illinois 60016
(312) 837-6973

Lowell Scott Weil
420 Lee Street
Des Plaines, Illinois 60016
(312) 837-6973

Frederick M. Weil
1601 Tanglewood
Hanover Park, Illinois 60103

William H. Harant
430 South Main Street
Lombard, Illinois 60148

Frederick H. Miller
325 West Prospect Avenue
Mt. Prospect, Illinois 60056

Gregory C. Bryniczka
7954 Oakton
Niles, Illinois 60648

John Durkin
365 East North Avenue
Northlake, Illinois 60164
(312) 345-8100

Gerald Quinlan
5405 West 95th Street
Oak Lawn, Illinois 60453
(312) 425-7476

George B. Geppner
4016 North Prospect Road
Peoria, Illinois 61614
(309) 685-5966

INDIANA

Raymond E. Stidd
2250 Midway Street
Columbus, Indiana 47201

Ronald L. Banta
4787 North Post Road
Indianapolis, Indiana 46226

Charles Walter Kelley III
1415 Shelby Street
Indianapolis, Indiana 46203
(317) 631-4011

Edward P. Morris
705 Jackson Street
La Porte, Indiana 46350

James P. Hoover
3420 State Road 26 East
Lafayette, Indiana 47905

KANSAS

Donald M. Miller
208 Wolcott Building
Hutchinson, Kansas 67501
(316) 665-5921

KENTUCKY

Robert G. Levine
9110 Leesgate Road
Louisville, Kentucky 40222
(502) 426-7222

MAINE

Roy B. Corbin
96 Harlow Street
Bangor, Maine 04401
(207) 825-3653

MARYLAND

Neil M. Scheffler
5205 East Drive
Arbutus, Maryland 21227

Paul L. Sheitel
5205 East Drive
Arbutus, Maryland 21227

Joseph D. Fox
9101 Franklin Square Drive
Baltimore, Maryland 20705
(301) 574-3900

Vito Nicholas Giardina
4115 Wilkens Avenue
Baltimore, Maryland 21229
(301) 242-7066

Steven M. Glubo
1001 Ingleside Avenue
Baltimore, Maryland 21228

John D. Freid
10518 Baltimore Boulevard
Beltsville, Maryland 20705

Edwin S. Hockstein
National Naval Medical Center
Bethesda, Maryland 20013

SHELDON P. KONECKE*
5530 Wisconsin Avenue, #835
Chevy Chase, Maryland 20015

Ronald A. Footer
615 South Frederick Avenue
Suite 304
Gaithersburg, Maryland 20760

Constantine Dimotisis
5953 Fisher Road, #101
Oxon Hill, Maryland 20031

Mark E. Landry
10500 South Glen Road
Potomac, Maryland 20854

Lanny Rubin
5310 Old Court Road
Randallstown, Maryland 21133

Raymond Merkin
11125 Rockville Pike
Rockville, Maryland 20852

MURRAY J. POLITZ*
121 Congressional Lane
Rockville, Maryland 20852

PAUL M. TAYLOR*
8630 Fenton Street
Silver Spring, Maryland 20910
(301) 587-5666

Lawrence D. Block
300 East Joppa Road
Towson, Maryland 21204

MASSACHUSETTS

Rob Roy McGregor
185 Pilgrim Road
Boston, Massachusetts 02215

Robert J. Scardina
185 Pilgrim Road
Boston, Massachusetts 02215
(617) 734-7000

Peter J. Barrett
Off 10 Martins Lane
Hingham, Massachusetts 02043

David B. Corn
252 South Huntington Avenue
Jamaica Plain, Massachusetts 02130

Arthur G. Swedlow
114 Waltham Street
Lexington, Massachusetts 02173

Kenneth I. Sann
103 Main Street
North Adams, Massachusetts 01247
(413) 663-5547

MICHIGAN

Barry D. Bean
19350 West 7 Mile
Detroit, Michigan 48219

Herbert Bean
19350 West 7 Mile
Detroit, Michigan 48219

Barry H. Galison
10573 Morang
Detroit, Michigan 48224
(313) 886-2355

Jerome Levine
18215 Joy Road
Detroit, Michigan 48228

David W. Ginsberg
2649 Clio Road
Flint, Michigan 48504

Herbert L. Kateman
282 South Irish Road
Flint, Michigan 48507

Terrance J. Emiley
6690 South Division Avenue
Grand Rapids, Michigan 49508

ALLYN E. PEELEN*
725 Alger, Southeast
Grand Rapids, Michigan 48507
(616) 245-5944

Rodney R. Senneker
66905 Division Avenue, S.E.
Grand Rapids, Michigan 49508

Charles R. Young
19075 Middlebelt Road
Livonia, Michigan 48152

Robert L. Lederman
36640 Gratiot Avenue
Mt. Clemens, Michigan 48043

Bruce M. Jacob
20960 Glenmorra
Southfield, Michigan 48076

Steven H. Glickman
5137 Rochester Road
Troy, Michigan 48084

Terry L. Freed
4230 East Ten Mile Road
Warren, Michigan 48091
(313) 758-5770

Robert N. Glick
13500 East 12 Mile Road
Warren, Michigan 48093

MINNESOTA

Fred G. Albert
408 Fourth Avenue, N.W.
P.O. Box 646
Austin, Minnesota 55912

Jerry D. Christenson
9050 Lyndale Avenue South
Bloomington, Minnesota 55420

MISSISSIPPI

Bruce Miller
962 Courthouse Road, Apt. 5
Gulfport, Mississippi 39501
(601) 626-6193

MISSOURI

C. Douglas De Tray
15605 East 24 Highway
Independence, Missouri 64050
(816) 461-3535

C. H. Wunderlich
118 East Jefferson
Kirkwood, Missouri 63122

Edward D. Stein
2428 Woodson Road
Overland, Missouri 63114

Jeffrey S. Brooks
4930 Lindell Boulevard
St. Louis, Missouri 63108

James L. Olroyd
4930 Lindell Boulevard
St. Louis, Missouri 63108

MONTANA

ROBERT L. PHILLIPS*
900 8th Avenue South
Great Falls, Montana 59405
(406) 761-2222

NEBRASKA

Michael J. Burns
811 Norris Avenue
McCook, Nebraska
(308) 345-3044

William L. McAvoy
401 East Gold Coast Road
Suite 326
Papillion, Nebraska 68046

NEW JERSEY

Charles H. Boxman
54 South Carolina Avenue
Atlantic City, New Jersey 08401
(609) 345-1696

Kenneth M. Koplow
141 South Black Hourse Pike
Blackwood, New Jersey 08012
(619) 228-1211

Joel Z. Zerinsky
466 Pompton Avenue
Cedar Grove, New Jersey 07009
(201) 857-1184

Jeffrey M. Cohen
142 Engle Street
Englewood, New Jersey 07631
(201) 568-0033

Norman J. Calihman
1555 Center Avenue
Fort Lee, New Jersey 07024

Franklin N. Levison
326 Cross Street, Apt 51
Fort Lee, New Jersey 07024
(201) 947-6163

William J. Accomando
6 Passaic Street
Hackensack, New Jersey 07601
(201) 488-7577

Morris R. Morin
6 Passaic Street
Hackensack, New Jersey 07601

Carmen A. Martina
319 10th Avenue
Haddon Heights, New Jersey 08035
(609) 546-6459

Leonard A. Zingler
245 Diamond-Bridge Avenue
Hawthorne, New Jersey 07506

Sophie Bakke
438 Broadway
Long Branch, New Jersey 07740

Theodore W. Jurgenson
438 Broadway
Long Branch, New Jersey 07740

GUIDO A. LA PORTA*
6 Heather Drive
Marlton, New Jersey 08053
(609) 983-6036

SANFORD WEINGER*
116 Millburn Avenue
Millburn, New Jersey 07041
(201) 376-3756

Robert E. Corso
54 Plymouth Street
Montclair, New Jersey 07042
(201) 744-9109

Nathan Sabin
44 Washington Street
Morristown, New Jersey 07960
(201) 538-4400

Norman M. Heifitz
1033 River Road
New Milford, New Jersey 07646

Walter Bennett
2113 River Road
Point Pleasant, New Jersey 08742
(201) 899-8140

George A. Sheehan, M.D.
79 West Front Street
Red Bank, New Jersey 07701
(201) 741-2027

Larry Price
636 Westwood Avenue
River Vale, New Jersey 07675
(201) 666-5115

David Plotkin
379 Meisel Avenue
Springfield, New Jersey 07081
(201) 379-9333

Andrew D. Dwyer
401 Shore Road
Somers Point, New Jersey 08244
(609) 927-4894

Myron A. Bergman
242 East Main Street
Somerville, New Jersey 08876
(201) 722-7872

Alan J. Greenberg
66 Sunset Strip
Succasunna, New Jersey 07876
(201) 584-1960

Richard F. Alfano
743 Estates Boulevard, Apt. #58
Trenton, New Jersey 08619

THOMAS M. MCGUIGAN*
One Highgate Drive
Suite B
Trenton, New Jersey 08618

John N. Spedick
2502 Nottingham Way
Trenton, New Jersey 08619
(609) 587-0707

Ronald Markizon
238 Chestnut Avenue
Vineland, New Jersey 08360
(609) 691-2152

John E. McNerney
490 Washington Avenue
Westwood, New Jersey 07675
(214) 221-2538

NEW MEXICO

Robert M. Parks
121 Sycamore, N.E.
Albuquerque, New Mexico 87106
(505) 247-4164

Donald E. Saye
1441 Wyoming Boulevard, N.E.
Albuquerque, New Mexico 87112
(505) 296-1882

Marc A. Stess
1405 Luisa, #2
Santa Fe, New Mexico 87501
(505) 988-8863

NEW YORK

Norbert B. Kosinski
504 Madison Avenue
Albany, New York 12208

Joseph F. Lalia
421 Deer Park Avenue
Babylon, New York 11702
(516) 587-9833

Saran A. Paul
42 Brentwood Road
Bayshore, New York 11706

James F. Hogan
41 Oak Street
Binghamton, New York 13905
(607) 723-7454

Dennis E. Shavelson
1604 Westchester Avenue
Bronx, New York 10472
(212) 991-3939

HARVEY STRAUSS*
2 West Fordham Road
Bronx, New York 10468

Lester Dennis
743 Manhattan Avenue
Brooklyn, New York 11222
(212) 389-4404

Gary J. Sherman
7902 Bay Parkway
Brooklyn, New York 11214

Bruce J. Bronstein
1725 Liberty Bank Building
Buffalo, New York 14202
(716) 856-5055

Anthony F. De Vincentis
1094 Love Joy Street
Buffalo, New York 14206

Edward H. Fischman
1431 Hertel Avenue
Buffalo, New York 14216
(716) 838-1131

Robert J. Rudewicz
3423 Bailey Avenue
Buffalo, New York 14215
(716) 836-8123

David M. Simon
2992 Bailey Avenue
Buffalo, New York 14215
(716) 832-2762

Edward M. Recoon
162 George Urban Boulevard
Cheektowaga, New York 14225
(716) 896-6262

Alan J. Sandler
Medical Executive Center
Clifton Park, New York 12065

RICHARD SCHUSTER*
1420 120th Street
College Point, New York 11356

SHELDON LANGER*
21E Industry Ct.
Deer Park, New York 11729

Karl Friedman
4 Cascade Ct.
Dix Hills, New York 11746

Leonard Light
614 Central Avenue
Dunkirk, New York 14048
(716) 366-6393

Arthur Robinson
159 E. 4th Street
Dunkirk, New York 14048
(716) 366-1170

Paul J. Maglione
275 Columbus Avenue
East White Plains, New York 10604
(914) 428-2743

Arthur S. Lukoff
77 North Main Street
Ellenville, New York 12428
(914) 647-3060

Mark A. Brenner
73-09 Myrtle Avenue
Glendale, New York 11227

Hyman H. Graver
179 Buffalo Street
Hamburg, New York 14075
(716) 649-2892

Russel K. Miller
146 Buffalo Street
Hamburg, New York 14075
(716) 649-1610

Jordan W. Rachlin
221 East Hartsdale Avenue
Hartsdale, New York 10530
(914) 472-9272

Richard M. Montag
380 Front Street
Suite 1E
Hempstead, New York 11550
(516) 483-7386

Jerome Sklar
84-39 153rd Avenue
Howard Beach, New York 11414
(212) 848-2000

Gary P. Milack
89-08 164th Street
Jamaica, New York 11432

Stephen P. Kaplan
90 Main Street
Kings Park, New York 11754

Stewart L. Rosensky
90 Main Street
Kings Park, New York 11754

Stephen A. Cutler
1271 Ridge Road
Lackawanna, New York 14218
(716) 824-9835

Bruce I. Dribbon
3000 Hempstead Turnpike
Levittown, New York 11756

Gordon Mittleman
Bewley Building
Suite 236
Lockport, New York 14094
(716) 433-6775

Robert N. Piccora
22 Crab Avenue
Lynbrook, New York 11563

Michael J. Valletta
Putnam Professional Park
Mahopac, New York 10541

Edwin J. Bruno
1600 Harrison Avenue
Mamaroneck, New York 10543
(914) 698-6863

Marc J. Hudes
267 Broadway
Monticello, New York 12701

Steven E. Baff
57 West 57th Street
New York, New York 10019
(212) 687-2851

Richard S. Bass
244 East 86th Street
New York, New York 10028
(212) 737-3374

Irving S. Buchbinder
53-55 East 124th Street
New York, New York 10035

Joe C. D'Amico
53 East 124th Street
New York, New York 10035

Joseph B. Dobrusin
25 Fifth Avenue
New York, New York 10003

Lewis Feinman
305 East 86th Street
New York, New York 10028

LOUIS C. GALLI*
9 East 96th Street
New York, New York 10028
(212) 348-6120

JOSEPH J. GELDWERT*
9 East 96th Street
New York, New York 10028
(213) 348-6120

Patrick M. Luongo
27 West 72nd Street
Suite 210
New York, New York 10023

Louis Shure
180 East End Avenue
New York, New York 10028

Monroe H. Tirnauer
4929 Broadway
New York, New York 10034
(212) 567-1252

Murray F. Weisenfeld
47 West 34th Street
New York, New York 10001

Ronald M. Werter
160 West End Avenue
New York, New York 10023

Phillip L. Whitman
319 East 50th Street
New York, New York 10022

Jay D. Helman
180 East Central Avenue
Pearl River, New York 10965
(914) 735-8440

Jeffrey A. Parker
123 Pike Street
Port Jervis, New York 12771
(914) 856-7700

Lewis J. Sims
69 West Cedar Street
Poughkeepsie, New York 12601
(914) 471-2243

Edward J. Stamm
69 West Cedar Street
Poughkeepsie, New York 12601
(914) 471-2243

Elliot B. Zacker
98-51 Queens Boulevard
Rego Park, New York 11374
(212) 897-3628

Eugene F. Gallagher
37 West Second Street
Riverhead, New York 11910
(516) 727-3592

Edward J. Bonavilla
490 Titus Avenue
Rochester, New York 14617

DAVID H. CONWAY*
368 South Goodman Street
Rochester, New York 14607

Paul Shevin
150 Theodore Fremel Avenue
Rye, New York 10580

Ronald Feldman
4100 Duff Place
Seaford, New York 11783
(516) 796-2900

JUSTIN WERNICK*
3921 Merrick Road
Seaford, New York 11783

Howard F. Baskin
263 North Main Street
Spring Valley, New York 10977

Steven L. Weinstein
2375 Richmond Road
Staten Island, New York 10306
(212) 979-1333

Neil R. Siegel
11 North Airmont Road
Suffern, New York 10901
(914) 357-4433

Donald A. Maron
713 East Genesee Street
Syracuse, New York 13210

Lee J. Carrel
107 Broad Street
Tonawanda, New York 14150

Dennis G. Winiecki
15 Webster Street
Tonawanda, New York 14120
(716) 692-2308

J. David Skliar
1825 Fifth Avenue
Troy, New York 12180
(518) 272-6881

Joel Cohen
1228 Wantagh Avenue
Wantagh, New York 11793
(516) 785-1505

Joel L. Spivack
One Strawberry Road
West Nyack, New York 10994
(914) 358-0500

Alvin J. Kanegis
146 A Post Street
Westbury, New York 11590
(516) 334-8208

Jeffrey M. Carrel
388 Evans Street
Williamsville, New York 14221

David M. Davidson
388 Evans Street
Williamsville, New York 14221

Kenneth T. Goldstein
388 Evans Street
Williamsville, New York 14221
(716) 634-9177

Christopher A. Orlando
260 South Broadway
Yonkers, New York 10705

NORTH CAROLINA

Richard D. Lotwin
888 East Franklin Street
Chapel Hill, North Carolina 27514
(919) 942-8878

Raymond E. Brown
4126 Park Road
Charlotte, North Carolina 28209
(704) 527-5724

Blair M. Bycura
401 South Marietta Street
Gastonia, North Carolina 28052
(704) 866-8521

Harvey G. Tilles
614 North Hamilton
P.O. Box 5466
High Point, North Carolina 27262
(919) 882-3021

J. BARRY JOHNSON*
301 Miller Street
Winston-Salem, North Carolina 27103

OHIO

Dixie A. Dooley
69 West Franklin Street
Centerville, Ohio 45459

Ronald C. Hetman
69 West Franklin Street
Centerville, Ohio 45459
(614) 433-0444

Rodney L. Tomczak
315 Solon Road
Chagrin Falls, Ohio 44022

Richard Steinberg
7225 Colerain Avenue
Cincinnati, Ohio 45239
(513) 521-7000

Nancy L. Conrad
1106 South Court Street
Circleville, Ohio 43113
(614) 474-3850

JOSEPH I. SEDER*
9500 Euclid Avenue
Cleveland, Ohio 44106
(216) 444-2200

Thomas Tauscheck
3760 Mayfield Road
Cleveland Heights, Ohio 44121
(216) 291-1903

Harry Zelwin
3237 De Sota
Cleveland Heights, Ohio 44121

John M. Norton
4355 North Hight Street
Columbus, Ohio 43214

Richard A. Raabe
1980 Mackenzie Drive
Columbus, Ohio 43220

David N. Wright
2680 North Haven Boulevard
Suite 5
Cuyahoga Falls, Ohio 44223
(216) 929-8641

Sheemon A. Wolfe
2422 Salem Avenue
Dayton, Ohio 45406

William M. Finerty
666 South Clinton Street
Defiance, Ohio 43512
(419) 782-2524

Thomas M. Hampton
1541 East 191 Street, K-349
Euclid, Ohio 44117
(216) 486-2938

W. Ray Bennett
922 Blanchard Avenue
Findlay, Ohio 45840

Gary L. Cramer
210 Baldwin Avenue
Findlay, Ohio 45840
(419) 932-0791

Karl J. Kaufman
4547 Mentor Avenue
Mentor, Ohio 44060

Robert C. Hoffecker
Milan Avenue Medical Center
Norwalk, Ohio 44857

Charles R. Marlow
1614 South Byrne Road
Toledo, Ohio 43614

OKLAHOMA

W. Bradley Johnston
2009 Barryton
Oklahoma City, Oklahoma 73120

OREGON

STEVEN ROY, M.D.*
Student Health Center
Oregon State University
Corvallis, Oregon 97331
(503) 754-2721

Ronald E. Walker
1585 SW Marlow Avenue
Suite 105
Portland, Oregon 97227

Raymond F. Hemphill
2418 Grear, N.E.
Salem, Oregon 97301
(503) 378-0056

John E. Hahn
11820 S.W. King James Place
Tigard, Oregon 97223
(503) 639-8107

Richard T. Dudzinski
2528 Sunset Boulevard
Houston, Texas 77005
(713) 522-5640

Marion J. Filippone
2041 West Alabama
Houston, Texas 77098
(713) 526-1441

Jonathan D. Hyman
442 Uvalde Road
Houston, Texas 77015
(713) 455-2384

Gary M. Lepow
4152 Bellaire Boulevard
Houston, Texas 77025

Ronald A. Robins
8762 Long Point
Houston, Texas 77055
(713) 461-1010

Ronald D. Sandler
909-P Federal Road
Houston, Texas 77015

WILLIAM L. VAN PELT*
1111 Geasner Road
Houston, Texas 77055

Ronald Bruscia
507 East 5th Street
Katy, Texas 77450

Michael Z. Metzger
1120 West Main Street
Lewisville, Texas 75067
(214) 221-2538

Charles A. Roberts
P.O. Box 754
Waxahachie, Texas 75165
(214) 937-1354

UTAH

H. Gary Morley
1275 North University Avenue, #12
Provo, Utah 94601
(801) 374-6900

VERMONT

Carl H. Kaczanowski
Executive Square
346 Shelburne Street
Burlington, Vermont 05401
(802) 658-0709

VIRGINIA

Jerome L. Dovberg
250 South Whiting Street
Alexandria, Virginia 22304

Myles J. Schneider
7420 Little River Turnpike
Annandale, Virginia 22003

Steven M. Yellin
1805 South Main Street
Blacksburg, Virginia 24060
(703) 951-8844

Raymond J. Olkin
10721 Main Street
Fairfax, Virginia 22030
(703) 273-3622

Charles J. Shuman
3545 Chain Bridge Road
Suite #1
Fairfax City, Virginia 22030

Raymond R. Alferink
1616A James Road (River Village)
Ft. Belvoir, Virginia 22060

Barry L. Swedlow
1938 Thompson Drive
Lynchburg, Virginia 24501

James H. Steinberg
13193 Warwich Boulevard
Newport News, Virginia 23802
(804) 877-6425

Paul M. Shoenfeld
707 South Jefferson Street
Suite 405
Roanoke, Virginia 24011
(703) 982-8722

Michael A. Robinson
613 Piney Branch Drive
Apt. 103
Virginia Beach, Virginia 23451

Arnold D. Levin
4225 Dale Boulevard
Woodbridge, Virginia 22193
(703) 670-9401

WASHINGTON

David W. Genuit
2528 Wheaton Way
Suite 105
Bremerton, Washington 98310
(206) 479-4060

Gerald T. Kuwada
401 South 43rd
Suite 130
Renton, Washington 98055
(206) 226-1780

ROBERT H. ARMSTRONG*
Safeco Plaza Tower
Seattle, Washington 98105
(206) 634-3344

Gary L. Dockery
1445 Medical Dental Building
509 Olive Way
Seattle, Washington 98101
(206) 623-6811

STANLEY G. NEWELL*
8523 15th NE
Seattle, Washington 98115
(206) 524-0771

Jack L. Morris
P.O. Box 552
Sunnyside, Washington 98944
(509) 837-4228

KURT BLAU*
1412 Medical Arts Building
Tacoma, Washington 98402
(206) 627-4181

Norton J. Schlesinger
209 South 12th Avenue
Yakima, Washington 98902

WEST VIRGINIA

Stephen R. Folickman
2917 University Avenue
Morgantown, West Virginia 26505
(304) 599-9000

WISCONSIN

Mark I. Julsrud
1836 South Avenue
La Crosse, Wisconsin 54601
(608) 782-2422

Edward R. Hommel
127 East Mifflin Street
Madison, Wisconsin 53703

Norman Mislove
6114 West Capitol Drive
Milwaukee, Wisconsin 53216
(414) 463-7330

Michael B. Thompson
2021 Washington Avenue
Racine, Wisconsin 53403
(414) 637-8806

CANADA

Kel Sherkin
75 The Donway West, #714
Don Mills, Ontario M3C 2E9,
    Canada
(609) 667-3785

David W. Weston
277 King Street West
Kitchner, Ontario, Canada

Shel Freelan
3415 Dixie
Missausaga, Ontario, Canada

James Brittain
47 Prince Street
Oshawa, Ontario L16 4C9, Canada
(416) 725-5621

David E. Greenberg
210 Gladstone
Ottawa, Ontario K2P 046, Canada
(613) 236-6246

Paul O'Connell
2100 Ellesmere Road, #206
Scarboro (Toronto), Ontario
    M1M3B7, Canada
(416) 431-6900

Lloyd I. Nesbitt
586 Eglinton Avenue E, #801
Toronto, Ontario M4P1P2, Canada
(416) 482-2230

Arnold M. Goldman
547 Eglinton Avenue
West Toronto M5 N 1B5
Ontario, Canada
(416) 485-4421

Alan M. Lustig
48 Leslie Street
Suite 306
Willowdale, Ontario, Canada
(416) 493-8144

Thomas A. Stevens
352 Sheppard Avenue East
Willowdale, Ontario M2N 3B4,
    Canada
(416) 223-9986

Raymond P. Tomaszewski
14 Hanna Street, East
Windsor, Ontario, Canada

*Please Note: All names with asterisks in FULL CAPITALS are Fellowship Members of the American Academy of Podiatric Sports Medicine who have met the requirements by passing the oral and written examination criteria in PODIATRIC SPORTS MEDICINE.

All other members listed are interested podiatrists not necessarily involved in sports medicine.

SOURCE: The American Academy of Podiatric Sports Medicine.

Appendix C
Where to Get a Stress Electrocardiogram

ALABAMA

L. T. Sheffield, M.D.
Cardiology Division
School of Medicine
University of Alabama
University Station
Birmingham, Alabama 35294
(205) 934-2274

T. Dye, M.D.
NASA Medical Center
Marshall Space Flight Center
Building 4249
Huntsville, Alabama 35815
(205) 453-2391

T. R. Figarola
Ambulatory Care Center
Universtiy of Alabama Medical
    School
Huntsville, Alabama
(205) 536-5511

ARKANSAS

B. S. Brown, M.D.
Department of Physical Education
Human Performance Laboratory
University of Arkansas
Fayetteville, Arkansas 72701
(501) 575-2859

John Boyce Davis, Ed.D.
CVR Fitness Clinic
University of Arkansas at Monticello
P.O. Box 2507
Monticello, Arkansas 71655
(501) 367-6811, Ext. 13

H. Orlee, Ed.D.
Exercise Physiology Laboratory
Box 765
Harding College
Searcy, Arkansas 72143
(501) 268-6161

CALIFORNIA

Director
CPR Center
Arcadia Methodist Hospital
300 West Huntington Drive
Arcadia, California 91006
(213) 445-4441

Director
CPR Center
Mercy Hospital
2215 Truxtun Avenue
Bakersfield, California 93301
(805) 327-3371

P. Schloemp
Central YMCA
2001 Allston Way
Berkeley, California 94707
(415) 848-6800

N. H. Mellor, M.D.
Cardiovascular Stress Test and
    Work Evaluation Unit
Circle City Hospital
730 Old Magnolia Avenue
Corona, California 91720
(714) 735-1211

Rudolph H. Dressendorder, Ph.D.
Adult Fitness Program
Department of Physical Education
University of California/Davis
Davis, California 95616
(916) 752-0511

Director
CPR Center
433 West Bastanchury Road
Fullerton, California 92635
(714) 870-9577

Director
CPR Center
Memorial Hospital
1420 South Central Avenue
Glendale, California 91204
(213) 246-6711

D. R. Fitch, M.D.
F. E. Gossard, M.D.
J. B. Maryland, M.D.
1808 Verdugo Boulevard
Glendale, California 91208
(213) 790-4631

Director
CPR Center
Antelope Valley Hospital
1600 West Avenue "J"
Lancaster, California 93534
(805) 948-4577

C. Ronald McBride, M.D.
Marina Medical Testing Center
4560 Admiralty Way
Marina del Rey, California 90291
(213) 823-7981

Director
CPR Center
Marina Mercy Hospital
4650 Lincoln Boulevard
Marina del Rey, California 90291
(213) 823-8911

Director
CPR Center
Mission Community Hospital
27802 Puerto Real Highway
Mission Viejo, California 92675
(714) 831-2300

Director
CPR Center
Riverside Hospital
12629 Riverside Drive
North Hollywood, California 91607
(213) 980-9200

Director
CPR Center
1215 West LaVeta
Suite 101
Orange, California 92668
(714) 997-1222

W. L. Haskell, Ph.D.
Division of Cardiology
Stanford Medical School
730 Welch Road
Palo Alto, California 94034
(415) 497-6254

L. Moskowitz, RNMS
Sequoia Hospital—YMCA CPR
Whipple and Alameda
Redwood City, California 94061
(415) 369-5811

J. L. Boyer, M.D.
Adult Physical Fitness Program
Exercise Laboratory
San Diego State University
San Diego, California 92115
(714) 287-2222

F. W. Kasch, Ph.D.
Adult Fitness Program
Physical Education Building
San Diego State University
San Diego, California 92182
(714) 286-5560

R. Martin
Aerobic Fitness Program
Downtown YMCA
1115 Eighth Avenue
San Diego, California 92101
(714) 323-7451

H. D. Peabody, Jr., M.D.
Department of Cardiology
Rees-Stealy Clinic
2001 Fourth Avenue
San Diego, California 92101
(714) 234-6261

B. H. McFadden M.D.
Santa Barbara Heart and Lung
    Institute
Galeta Valley Hospital
351 Patterson Avenue
Santa Barbara, California 93111
(805) 967-3411

Steven M. Kaye, M.D.
2416 B. Castillo Street
Santa Barbara, California 93205
(805) 964-1582

T. D. Gardiner, M.D.
18740 Ventura Boulevard
Tarzana, California 91356
(213) 881-2232

Director
South Bay CPR Center
22352 Hawthorne Boulevard
Torrance, California 90505
(213) 373-6769

E. P. Cafdello, M.D.
YMCA Exercise Testing Program
4201 Torrance Boulevard
Suite 360
Torrance, California 90503
(213) 540-5522

Director
CPR Center
Whittier Hospital
15151 Janine Drive
Whittier, California 90605
(213) 945-3561

COLORADO

B. Balke, M.D.
Aspen Cardiopulmonary
    Rehabilitation Unit
Box 630
Aspen, Colorado 81611
(303) 925-1992

G. P. Smith, Director
Cardiac Reconditioning
Hilltop House
515 Patterson Avenue
Grand Junction, Colorado 81501
(303) 242-2801

DELAWARE

Director
Cardiac and Pulmonary
104 Hagley Building
Concord Plaza
3411 Silverside Road
Wilmington, Delaware 19810
(302) 478-7930

WASHINGTON, D.C.

S. M. Fox, III, M.D.
Cardiology Exercise Laboratory
Georgetown University
3800 Reservoir Road, N.W.
Washington, D.C. 20007
(202) 625-2001

J. R. Snyder, M.D.
Washington Cardiovascular
    Rehabilitation Center
916 Nineteenth Street, N.W.
Washington, D.C. 20066
(202) 541-4666

FLORIDA

J. Esterson, M.D.
2526 E. Hallandale Beach Boulevard
Hallandale, Florida 33009
(305) 456-5115

Director
CPR Center
Mercy Professional Building
Suite 2
3661 South Miami Avenue
Miami, Florida 33133
(305) 854-0982

H. Gilmore
Pankey Dental Institute
DuPont Plaza Hotel
Miami, Florida 33131
(305) 371-8711

Director
Cardiac Rehabilitation Unit
Florida Hospital
601 East Rollins Street
Orlando, Florida 32803
(305) 896-6611

Z. C. Burton, Jr., M.D.
500 East Colonial Drive
Orlando, Florida 32803
(305) 841-7151

Director
CPR Center
1717 North "E" Street
P.O. Box 19036
Pensacola, Florida 32503
(904) 434-4666

GEORGIA

J. D. Cantwell, M.D.
Preventive Cardiology Clinic
433 Highland Avenue, N.E.
Atlanta, Georgia 30312
(404) 524-3633

J. D. Cantwell, M.D.
G. F. Fletcher, M.D.
Cardiology Division
Georgia Baptist Hospital
300 Boulevard, N.E.
Atlanta, Georgia 30312
(404) 659-4211

C. A. Gilbert, M.D.
Cardiac Function Laboratory
Grady Memorial Hospital
69 Butler Street, S.E.
Atlanta, Georgia 30303
(404) 588-4307

HAWAII

J. Schaff, Jr., M.D.
Cardiac Rehabilitation Program
Central YMCA
401 Atkinson Drive
Honolulu, Hawaii 96814
(808) 941-3344

ILLINOIS

R. G. Knowlton, Ph.D.
Adult Fitness Program
Department of Physical Education
Southern Illinois University
Carbondale, Illinois 62801
(618) 453-2575

Director
CPR Center
Galesburg Cottage Hospital
695 North Kellogg Street
Galesburg, Illinois 61401
(309) 343-8131

N. D. Nequin, M.D.
Physiological Performance Laboratory
Leaning Tower YMCA
6300 West Touhy Avenue
Niles, Illinois 60648
(312) 647-8222

Director
CPR Center
Rock Island Franciscan Hospital
2701 Seventeenth Street
Rock Island, Illinois 61201
(309) 793-1000

R. R. Jirka, Ph.D.
Cardiovascular Rehabilitation
  and Prevention
YMCA of Madison County
Twelfth and Jackson
P.O. Box 231
Anderson, Indiana 46015
(317) 644-7796

N. Tremble, Ph.D.
Cardiovascular Fitness Clinic
Department of Physical Education
Drake University
Des Moines, Iowa 50311
(515) 271-2866

Director
CPR Center
Providence–St. Margaret Hospital
759 Vermont Avenue
Kansas City, Kansas 66101
(913) 621-0700

W. H. Osness, Ph.D.
Department of Physical Education
108 Robinson
University of Kansas
Lawrence, Kansas 66044
(913) 864-3371

R. G. McAlister, Jr., M.D.
Cardiology Division
Veterans Administration Hospital
Lexington, Kentucky 40507

YMCA Physical Fitness Network
936 St. Charles Avenue
New Orleans, Louisiana 70130
(504) 568-YMCA

Director
Maryland General Hospital
827 Linden Avenue
Baltimore, Maryland 21201
(301) 728-7900

Jack P. Segal, M.D.
5530 Wisconsin Avenue
Chevy Chase, Maryland 20015
(301) 656-9070

D. L. Santa Maria, Ed.D.
Sports Medicine and Physical
  Fitness Center
University of Maryland
College Park, Maryland 20742
(301) 454-4750

Director
CPR Center
Memorial Hospital
Memorial Avenue
Cumberland, Maryland 21502
(301) 777-4000

Director
CPR Center
Fallston General Hospital
200 Milton Avenue
Fallston, Maryland 21047
(301) 877-3700

The Sportsmedicine Institute
9900 Georgia Avenue
Silver Spring, Maryland 20902
(301) 589-0599

K. M. Lindgren, M.D.
Department of Cardiology
Washington Adventist Hospital
7600 Carroll Avenue
Takoma Park, Maryland 20012
(301) 891-7672

Director
CPR Center
Faulkner Health Care
780 American Legion Highway
Roslindale, Massachusetts 02131
(617) 325-1000

Director
CPR Center
St. Joseph's Hospital
302 Kensington Avenue
Flint, Michigan 48502
(313) 238-2601

Dr. Thomas J. Clay
308 Medical Arts Building
26 Sheldon Avenue, S.E.
Grand Rapids, Michigan 49503
(616) 451-3021

G. Schultz, P.E.D.
R. Parr, Ed.D.
J. Roitman. Ed.D.
J. Pauliski
Adult Fitness Program
Central Michigan University
Mount Pleasant, Michigan 48858
(517) 774-3580

R. J. Stewart, D.O.
Macomb Cardiac Rehabilitation
40600 Van Dyke
Sterling Heights, Michigan 48087
(313) 939-1313

J. Arends, M.D.
1551 West Big Beaver Road
Troy, Michigan 48084
(313) 643-7770

Mark Crooks, Ph.D.
Cardiovascular Rehabilitation
  Institute
6724 Troost
Suite 108
Kansas City, Missouri 64131

K. Berg, Ed.D.
W. Gust, M.D.
Department of Physical Education
6100 Dodge
University of Nebraska/Omaha
Omaha, Nebraska 68601
(402) 554-2670

Director
CPR Center
Sunrise Hospital
3186 Maryland Parkway
Las Vegas, Nevada 89109
(702) 735-2789

Stephen Dow, M.D.
Nevada Heart Fitness Institute
c/o The Athlete's Foot
580 North McCarran Boulevard
Sparkes, Nevada 89431
(702) 331-3145

NEW JERSEY

D. J. Henderson, Ph.D.
Stress Testing
56 Haddon Avenue
Haddonfield, New Jersey 08033
(609) 795-2220

I. M. Levitas, M.D.
Bergen County Heart Association
    Program—Hackensack Hospital
Hackensack, New Jersey 07601
(201) 487-4000 Ext. 383

E. M. Stein, M.D.
Memorial General Hospital
Stress Testing Laboratory
1000 Galloping Hill Road
Union, New Jersey 07083
(201) 964-5757

George Sheehan, M.D.
Stress Testing Program
Riverview Hospital
Red Bank, New Jersey 07701
(201) 741-2700

Director
Cardiology Section
St. Francis Medical Center
601 Hamilton Avenue
Trenton, New Jersey 08629
(609) 369-7676

NEW MEXICO

H. A. Atterbom, Ph.D.
Human Performance Laboratory
Johnson Gymnasium
University of New Mexico
Albuquerque, New Mexico 87131
(505) 277-4441

NEW YORK

Director
Victory Memorial Hospital
Brooklyn, New York 11228
(516) 422-1000

V. N. Smodlaka, M.D.
Rehabilitation Medicine Department
Methodist Hospital
506 Sixth Street
Brooklyn, New York 11215
(212) 780-3266

R. M. Kohn, M.D.
50 High Street
Suite 1104
Buffalo, New York 14203
(716) 885-2400

W. J. Tomik, Ph.D.
Physical Fitness and Heart
    Disease Intervention
State University College
Cortland, New York 13045
(607) 753-4944

Director
Central Nassau CPR
1900 Hempstead Turnpike
East Meadow, New York 11756
(516) 794-9797

M. McCain
Cardiovascular Testing and Exercise
    Program
Central Queens YMCA
89-25 Parsons Boulevard
Jamaica, New York 11432
(212) 739-6600

Director
EKG Department
CPR Center
Phelps Memorial Hospital
North Broadway
North Tarrytown, New York 10541
(914) 631-5100

Director
Manhattan CPR Center
211 East 51st Street
New York, New York 10022
(212) 371-6281

David Alderson
West Side YMCA
5 West 63rd Street
New York, New York 10023
(212) 787-4562

W. S. Gualtiere, Ph.D.
A. J. Delmoa, M.D.
Cardio-Metrics Institute
295 Madison Avenue
New York, New York 10017
(212) 889-6123

Alan S. Rosenberg, M.D.
1025 Northern Boulevard
Roslyn, New York 11576
(516) 627-8888

Director
Staten Island Diagnostic and
    Rehabilitation Center
11 Ralph Place
Staten Island, New York 10304
(212) 727-4900

NORTH CAROLINA

P. Ribisl, Ph.D.
Cardiac Rehabilitation Program
Human Performance Laboratory
Department of Physical Education
Wake Forest University
Winston-Salem, North Carolina
    27109
(919) 761-5394

OHIO

T. J. White
Downtown Canton YMCA
405 Second Street, N.W.
Canton, Ohio 44702
(216) 455-1536

T. E. Donaldson
Exercise Testing Laboratory
Central YMCA
2200 Prospect Avenue
Cleveland, Ohio 44115
(216) 696-2200

C. Long II, M.D.
Cardiac Evaluation and
    Rehabilitation Program
Highland View Hospital
3901 Ireland Drive
Cleveland, Ohio 44122
(216) 464-9600

S. W. Weinberg, M.D.
Cardiac Treatment Center
Good Samaritan Hospital
Dayton, Ohio
(513) 278-2612

Dr. Wayne Sinning
Applied Physiology Research
    Laboratory
Kent State University
Kent, Ohio 44242
(216) 672-2859

R. L. Miller, M.D.
Comprehensive Executive Health
    Evaluations
Executive Health Maintenance
    Programs
5335 Far Hills Avenue
Kettering, Ohio 45459
(513) 435-0220

Director
CPR Center
Lima Memorial Hospital
Linden and Mobel Streets
Lima, Ohio 45804
(419) 225-5967

Director
CPR Center
Mercy Hospital
1248 Kinneys Lane
Portsmouth, Ohio 45662
(614) 353-2131

W. J. Rowe, M.D.
Exercise Stress Testing
St. Vincent's Hospital
2213 Cherry Street
Toledo, Ohio 43608
(419) 259-4167

OKLAHOMA

Director
CPR Center
St. John's Hospital
1923 South Utica Avenue
Tulsa, Oklahoma 74104
(918) 744-2345

OREGON

Henry B. Garrison, M.D.
CAPRI
7645 South West Capital Highway
Portland, Oregon 97219
(543) 245-2291

W. A. Ray
Portland YMCA Cardiovascular
  Health Program
2831 S. W. Barbur Boulevard
Portland, Oregon 97201
(503) 223-9622

M. W. Tichy, Ph.D.
Adult Fitness Program
Portland State University
P.O. Box 751
Portland, Oregon 97207
(503) 229-4989

PENNSYLVANIA

Director
CPR Center
Allentown Sacred Heart Hospital
1200 South Cedarcrest Boulevard
Allentown, Pennsylvania 18103
(215) 821-2121

S. E. Zeeman, M.D.
901 North Nineteenth Street
Allentown, Pennsylvania 18104
(215) 437-5505

Director
CPR Center
Maple Avenue Hospital
Maple Avenue
DuBois, Pennsylvania 15801
(814) 371-3440

H. Weber, Ph.D.
Adult Fitness and Heart Evaluation
Koehler Field House
East Stroudsburg State College
East Stroudsburg, Pennsylvania 18301
(717) 424-3336

Director
CPR Center
2024 Lehigh Street
Easton, Pennsylvania 18042
(215) 252-0301

Director
CPR Center
Hamot Medical Center
201 State Street
Erie, Pennsylvania 16512
(814) 455-6711

Director
CPR Center
Medical Arts Building, Room 208
225 West 25th Street
Erie, Pennsylvania 16502
(814) 453-5485

Doctors Osteopathic Hospital
252 West 11th Street
Erie, Pennsylvania 16501
(814) 455-3961

Central Branch YMCA
Front and North Street
Harrisburg, Pennsylvania 17101
(717) 234-6221

Director
CPR Center
Northwestern Building
Suite 1108-1110
Hazelton, Pennsylvania 18201
(717) 455-9070

Ronald Legum, M.D.
CPR Center
St. Joseph's Hospital
250 College Avenue
Lancaster, Pennsylvania 17604
(717) 291-8291

Director
CPR Center
Spencer Hospital
1034 Grove Street
Meadville, Pennsylvania 16335
(814) 724-6622

Director
CPR Center
4950 Wilson Lane
Mechanicsburg, Pennsylvania 17055
(717) 697-8350

Director
CPR Center
JFK Memorial Hospital
Cheltenham Avenue and
  Langdon Street
Philadelphia, Pennsylvania 19124
(215) 289-6000

G. Berger
Physical Fitness Program
Central Branch YMCA
1421 Arch Street
Philadelphia, Pennsylvania 19102

N. Makous, M.D.
Cardiology Department
Pennsylvania Hospital
829 Spruce Street
Philadelphia, Pennsylvania 19107
(215) 829-3000

L. N. Adler, M.D.
Cardiac Rehabilitation Institute
532 South Aiken Avenue, No. 108
Pittsburgh, Pennsylvania 15232
(412) 682-6201

B. J. Robertson, Ph.D.
Human Laboratory
Department of Health and
  Physical Education
Universtiy of Pittsburgh
242 Tress Hall
Pittsburgh, Pennsylvania 15261
(412) 624-4387

Director
CPR Center
748 Quincey Avenue
Scranton, Pennsylvania 18510
(717) 961-3090

Director
CPR Center
Sharon General Hospital
740 East State Street
Sharon, Pennsylvania 16146
(412) 981-1700

E. R. Buskirk, Ph.D.
Laboratory for Human
  Performance Research
College of Health, Physical
  Education, and Recreation
Pennsylvania State University
University Park, Pennsylvania 16802
(814) 865-3453

Director
CPR Center
Mercy Hospital
196 Hanover Street
Wilkes-Barre, Pennsylvania
(717) 822-8101 Stress Lab

Director
CPR Center
924 C. Colonial Avenue
York, Pennsylvania 17403

SOUTH CAROLINA

P. C. Gazes, M.D.
Cardiovascular Division
Medical University Hospital
171 Ashley Avenue
Charleston, South Carolina 29403
(803) 792-3355

S. N. Blair, P.E.D.
Human Performance Laboratory
College of Physical Education
University of South Carolina
Columbia, South Carolina 29205
(803) 777-3890

YMCA Family Center
Bob Gilbertson
266 S. Pine Street
Spartanburg, South Carolina 29302
(803) 585-0306

TEXAS

K. H. Cooper, M.D.
Institute for Aerobics Research
12100 Preston Road
Dallas, Texas 75230
(214) 239-7223

John C. Holland, P.E.D.
Department of HPE
University of Houston
Houston, Texas 77004
(713) 749-4386

J. Quiocho
Physical Conditioning and
    Evaluation
YMCA
701 Montana Avenue
El Paso, Texas 79902
(915) 533-3941

D. Cardus, M.D.
Cardiac Rehabilitation
Texas Institute for Rehabilitation
    and Research
P.O. Box 20095
Texas Medical Center
Houston, Texas 77002
(713) 797-1440

A. K. Johnson
Houston Downtown YMCA
1600 Louisiana
Houston, Texas 77002
(713) 659-8501

UTAH

H. W. Buckner
YMCA
737 East Second South
Salt Lake City, Utah 84102
(801) 322-1291

VIRGINIA

F. Anderson, M.D.
Cardiology Department
Northern Virginia Doctors Hospital
601 Carlin Springs Road
Arlington, Virginia 22204
(703) 671-1200

R. F. Dietz, Jr., M.D.
Cardiac Laboratory
Arlington Hospital
Arlington, Virginia 22205
(703) 558-6267

G. E. Hahn, M.D.
Department of Cardiology
Prince William Hospital
8700 Sudley Road
Manassas, Virginia 22110
(703) 368-8121

WASHINGTON

W. Mead, M.D.
Universal Testing Services
8118 Greenlake Drive North
Seattle, Washington 98103
(206) 523-4700

H. R. Pyfer, M.D.
Cardio-Pulmonary Research
    Institute (CAPRI)
914 East Jefferson Street
Seattle, Washington 98122
(206) 323-7550

CAPRI
Green River College
So. Seattle, Wahington 98002
(206) 323-7550

D. Ballew, M.D.
Yakima Heart Center
302 South Tenth Avenue
Yakima, Washington 98901
(509) 248-7715

WISCONSIN

P. K. Wilson, Ed.D.
Cardiac Rehabilitation Program
University of Wisconsin/LaCrosse
Mitchell Hall
1820 Pine Street
LaCrosse, Wisconsin 54601
(608) 785-8684

R. J. Corliss, M.D.
F. Nagel, Ph.D.
Biodynamics Laboratory
University of Wisconsin
2000 Observatory Drive
Madison, Wisconsin 53706
(608) 262-9905

Director
CPR Center
Lutheran Hospital
2200 West Kilbourn Avenue
Milwaukee, Wisconsin 53233
(414) 344-8800

Index

carbohydrate depletion (diet), 42
carbohydrate packing, 41–44
carbon dioxide, 46, 47
cardiovascular fitness, 9–10, 95
Carr, Austin, 56
Carter, Don, 101
cartilage, 95, 111–112, 113, 135
Cashman, Wayne, 121
Castagnola, Lou, 79, 187
Castenada, Ted, 45
Castle, William, 76
casts, 110, 111, 112, 176–177
Causeret, J., 64
Cauthen, Steve, 5
Cavanaugh, Terrence, 21
cells, 51, 119, 155, 157
cellulose, 52
Cerutty, Percy, 83
Challant, Frank, 117, 146
Chamberlain, Wilt, 12
chest pain: angina, 22, 59; heart attack
    and, 20; non-heart attack, 20, 21,
    43
Chicago Black Hawks, 9, 31
Chittenden, Russell, 65
cholesterol, 50, 57, 58–60
Christenson, Erik, 40
chromium, 77, 78
circulation, and background training,
    35. See also cardiovascular fitness
Clancy, Gil, 65, 66
Clarke, Bobby, 34, 72
Clarke, Ron, 35
Clayton, Derek, 32–33, 46
clotting, 79. See also blood clots
clothing, 125, 166, 182–184; for cold-
    weather exercise, 158, 159–161, 162;
    for hot-weather exercise, 125, 145,
    149. See also hats; shoes; shorts;
    socks
cobalt, 77, 78
cocaine, 85
Cohn, Clarence, 64
colds, as sign of overtraining, 33
cold-weather exercise, 14, 40, 158–166,
    183
collateral circulation, 19, 20
Collins, Doug, 114, 135
colon, 104, 105
commercial beverages, 69, 82, 148–
    149
compression, as treatment. See RICE
conditioning: and digestion, 66; for hot
    weather, 144–145; for cold weather,
    158–159, 162; and injury recovery
    time, 95
Coney Island Polar Bears, 165
congestive heart failure, 21. See also
    heart attack; heart disease
Conners, Jimmy, 5
Consolazio, Frank, 65
constipation, as sign of overtraining,
    33
convulsions, 155, 157
Cooper, Donald L., 69, 169

Cooper, Kenneth, 20, 22, 81
coordination, training for, 28–29
copper, 50, 77, 78
cortisone, and cortisone injections, 101,
    118, 128, 135, 176
Costill, David, 45, 48, 51, 80
Counsilman, Doc, 29, 31–32, 34, 36,
    37, 66, 68, 69, 146
Counsilman, Marjorie, 49
Cowens, Dave, 135
cramps: menstrual, 15, 17; muscle,
    102–105; stomach, 65–66, 68, 148
Crawford, Jack, 51
Csonka, Larry, 4
Cureton, Tom, 16
curvature of the spine. See spine,
    curvature of
Cushmac, George, 152
cyanocobalamine. See vitamins, B₁₂

Dallas Tornado, 102
Darman, Jeff, 10
Davey, Tim, 71, 130, 139
Daws, Ron, 144–145, 147
Decker, Mary, 51
dehydration, 51, 78, 153, 154–155,
    156, 157, 162
DeMar, Clarence, 11–12, 182
depletion (training method), 40–41
depression, 24, 33, 87, 180. See also
    mood change
dermatologists, 122, 123, 127
de Vries, Herbert A., 16, 24, 46
dextromoramide, 85
diabetes, 15, 74
diagnosis, incorrect, of athletes by non-
    sportsmedicine physicians, 172–175
diaphragm, 103–105, 147
diarrhea, 33, 73, 82
Dickinson, L., 174
diet, 49–69, 104; calcium and, 82; for
    cold weather, 161–162; for hot
    weather, 146–149, 155–157 passim;
    liquid meals, 69; magnesium and,
    81–82; minerals and, 78, 82–83;
    myths about, 12–13; number of
    meals per day, 64; potassium and,
    80, 81; pre-competition, 65–69; salt
    and, 78, 79–80; vitamins and, 12,
    71–76. See also diets (specific);
    minerals; protein; vegetarian diet;
    vitamins
diethylamphetamine, 85
diets (specific): Carbohydrate Packing
    Diet, 43; 1,530 Carbohydrate Deple-
    tion Diet Plan, 42; Four-Food Plan,
    54–55; 4,355 Calorie Training Diet,
    60; Vegetarian (3,000 Calorie), 56
digestion, and exercise, 15, 24, 65–66,
    67, 68, 69
dimethylamphetamine, 85
Dionne, Marcel, 5
dipipanone, 85
disaccharides, 51. See also sugar

diuretics, 17, 51, 80
dizziness, 85, 92, 153, 154
dogs, and runners, 187
Drake, Lloyd, 34
Drescher, Dick, 90
drug control and testing, in profes-
    sional sports, 85, 86, 88, 91
drugs, 73, 74, 84–92. See also specific
    drugs
Druit, Guy, 155
drying agents, 122, 123
Dundee, Angelo, 9, 30, 33, 72

East Germany, sportsmedicine in, 7,
    34
"easy days," in training, 10–11, 27, 30,
    31, 187–194 passim. See also "hard
    days"
eating, rules for proper, 50–55, 104.
    See also diet
Edelen, Buddy, 145
Ekbloom, Bjorn, 47–48
elbow, 99, 112, 114. See also elbow
    tendonitis; tennis elbow
elbow tendonitis, 107
electrocardiograms: of athletes, 12,
    175; resting (vs. stress), 12; stress,
    12, 21, 181, 182, 213–218
elevation, as treatment. See RICE
Ellestand, Myrvin, 21
Elliot, Herb, 83
Emmerton, Bill, 181
endurance, 29, 34–35, 37, 39, 40, 47–
    48, 99, 187–194 passim
energy production, 40, 51–52, 61, 64,
    65, 81
ephedrine, 84, 85
Epsom salts. See magnesium
Erving, Julius ("Dr. J"), 4
Esposito, Phil, 5, 68
ethylamphetamine, 85
Evans, Herbert M., 75
evaporation, 80, 144–145, 149. See
    also sweat and sweating
Evert, Chris, 5, 138
Ewbank, Weeb, 169
excessive pronation. See pronation,
    excessive
exercise, benefits and popularity of, 3–
    4, 15–26, 128; effectiveness of vari-
    ous types rated, 181; during recovery
    from injury, 95, 96, 100, 107, 111.
    See also cardiovascular fitness; cold-
    weather exercise; exercises (specif-
    ic); hot-weather exercise; jogging;
    marathon running and marathons;
    running; sexual activity; training;
    warm-ups
exercises (specific): bent-knee sit-ups,
    105, 115; board stand, 109; for ilio-
    psoas muscle, 137; Japanese split,
    116, 140; leg extensions, 114; low-
    back stretch, 116; for shin splints,
    142; strengthening hamstrings, 140,
    141; strengthening knee muscles,

114; strengthening ligaments, 114; tennis elbow prevention, 102; toe touch, 116, 140; wall push-ups, 108, 116, 140. *See also* running; stretching

extreme temperatures, 14, 79, 144–166

fartlek, 191–192
fascia, 95, 117, 118, 119, 129, 133, 159
fasciitis. *See* plantar fasciitis
fast twitch fibers (muscle), 29
fatigue, 33, 81, 85, 92. *See also* conditioning; heat exhaustion
fats, 23, 25–26, 39, 41, 42, 50, 52, 54, 55, 57–60, 63–64, 65, 68, 92, 159, 171. *See also* diet
feet, 110, 111, 117, 118, 119; excessive pronation of, 114, 118, 133–134, 136, 182; high-arched, 133, 135, 136. *See also* arch supports; athlete's foot; blisters; orthotics; plantar fasciitis; plantar warts; shoes; socks
fencamfamin, 85
fertility, 73, 75, 90
fitness. *See* exercise
"flat feet." *See* pronation, excessive
flexibility, lack of, and injuries, 98, 129, 138–139. *See also* stretching
fluids, 27, 42, 46, 47, 50, 51, 65–69; and hot-weather exercise, 147–149, 152, 154, 155–157 *passim. See also* dehydration
fluorine, 78
folic acid, 78
food, basic groups, 50–53. *See also* carbohydrates; diet; diets (specific); fats; fluids; calories; minerals; protein; vitamins
forehand tennis elbow. *See* tennis elbow
Four-Food Plan, 54–55
Fox, Ted, 112
fractures, bone, 73, 133; complete, 109–110; stress, 109, 110–111
Frary, Mike, 175
freezing, 159
frostbite, 158, 162, 163–165
fructose, 51, 68
fungus, 122, 123

Gable, Dan, 9, 31, 65, 66, 80, 146
galactose, 51, 104
Galento, Tony, 68
Galloway, Jeff, 45
Gamble, James, 78–79
Gamble, Oscar, 4
gangrene, 164
gas, and cramps, 104
Geis, Paul, 45
Gibson, Bob, 101
Gilbert, Bill, 150
glomerulus, 174
gloves. *See* mittens
glucose, 51, 52, 67, 68

glutin, 104
glycogen, 13, 31, 39, 40–41, 43, 44, 45, 46, 47, 52, 187–188
Godfrey, William, 80
goiters, 83
Gonzales, Pancho, 101
Goodwin, Fred, 17, 18
Gordon, Gary, 114, 135
Gordonoff, T., 74
Gorilla Council of Nutrition, 73
Gorman, Pat, 22
Gossage, Rich, 5
Gottlieb, David G., 24
Greenberg, Leon A., 64
Greenwood, Robert, 18
Gregory, Dick, 72
Griese, Bob, 4
Greist, John H., 18
Griffith, Emil, 65

habit-forming drugs, distinguished from addiction, 86. *See also* addiction; amphetamines; vitamins
Haggard, Howard W., 64
Hamill, Dorothy, 26
hamstring, 138, 139–141, 189. *See also* hamstring pull
hamstring pull, 95, 100, 128–129, 139–141
hands, stress fractures in, 110
Hannus, Matti, 48
"hard days," in training, 10–11, 27, 30, 131, 187–194 *passim. See also* "easy days"
Hatch, Roy, 14, 158, 161
hats, 149–150, 161, 183
Havlicek, John, 117
Hawkins, Connie, 56
Haywood, Spencer, 142
headache, 15, 44, 85, 86, 157
heart, 23, 65–66, 86, 145, 146, 168, 181; of athletes, 11, 21, 175; and exercise, 9–10, 11–12, 19–22, 30–31, 35, 45, 95, 187. *See also* angina; heart attack; heart disease
heart attack, 11–12, 15, 19–20, 20–22, 52, 57, 59, 60–61, 62, 79, 92, 146
heart disease, 15, 21–22, 54, 57. *See also* angina; heart attack
heat: muscle, 77, 81, 147; and running, 150–152; to treat injuries, 99 (*See also* RICE). *See also* cold-weather exercise; hot-weather exercise; heat exhaustion; heatstroke
heat cramps. *See* cramps, muscle
heat exhaustion, 14, 79, 151, 154–157
heatstroke, 85, 87, 146, 150, 152–154; EMERGENCY TREATMENT, 154
heavy-leggedness, 33, 43, 44
Hedburg, Ander, 5
heel, 105, 117, 118. *See also* heel spurs
heel spurs, 118, 128
Hellerstein, Herman, 22
hemoglobin, 77, 173, 174

Henderson, Joe, 134
hepatitis, 92
heroin, 85
Hervey, G. H., 90
Hicks, Tom, 32
high-arched feet. *See* feet
high blood pressure, 14, 15
Hill, Ron, 41
hip, 112, 133, 135, 137, 140
Hisle, Larry, 4
"hitting the wall," 40–41, 160. *See also* "bonking"
Holloszy, John, 20, 37
"Holyoke Massacre" (marathon), 144–145, 146
Honolulu Marathon, 21
hostility, and amphetamines, 86. *See also* aggression
hot-weather exercise, 40, 79–80, 85, 103, 144–158, 183
Howard, Dick, 87
Hultman, Eric, 42
humidity, 151, 152, 154
hyperactivity, and amphetamine, 86
hyperthermia, 39
hyperventilating, and muscle cramps, 103
hypoglycemia, 39, 60. *See also* "rebound hypoglycemia"
hypothermia, 158, 162, 165–166
hypoxia, 39

ice, as treatment. *See* RICE
iliopsoas muscle, 115, 137
imbalance, muscle. *See* muscle imbalance
indomethacin, 126
infection, 34, 94, 110, 119, 121, 122, 123
inflammation of tendon. *See* tendonitis
injections, 13, 75, 76, 176. *See also* cortisone
injuries, 8–9, 33, 35, 80, 86, 87, 93–143, 186, 188–189, 190, 191
insomnia, 15, 17–18. *See also* sleep
Institute of Aerobic Research, 20
insulin, 60, 67, 77
intensity of exercise, 131, 132, 142–143. *See also* "easy days"; "hard days"; overtraining
interval technique (running), 29, 191–194 *passim*
intestine, 51, 85, 92, 104, 105
International Federation of Sports and Medicine, 91
iodine, 50, 77, 78, 83
iron poisoning, 73

Jackson, Reggie, 5, 138
Jacobs, Franklin, 10
Japanese split (exercise), 116, 140
Jascourt, Hugh, 151
Jenner, Bruce, 33
"jock itch," 123
jogging, 3, 18, 22, 41, 180–181, 184–185, 187, 189–194 *passim*